D0042049

eat dirt

eat dirt

Why Leaky Gut May Be the Root
Cause of Your Health Problems and
5 Surprising Steps to Cure It

DR. JOSH AXE

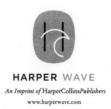

HARPER WAVE

An Imprint of HarperCollinsPublishers

www.harperwave.com

EAT DIRT. Copyright © 2016 by Dr. Josh Axe. All rights reserved. Printed in the United States of America. No part of this book may be used or reproduced in any manner whatsoever without written permission except in the case of brief quotations embodied in critical articles and reviews. For information, address HarperCollins Publishers, 195 Broadway, New York, NY 10007.

HarperCollins books may be purchased for educational, business, or sales promotional use. For information, please e-mail the Special Markets Department at SPsales@harpercollins.com.

FIRST EDITION

Designed by Jaime Putorti

Library of Congress Cataloging-in-Publication Data has been applied for.

ISBN: 978-0-06-243364-0

16 17 18 19 20   OV/RRD   10 9 8 7 6 5 4 3 2 1

I dedicate this book to Axe Nation, those courageous warriors who stand with me and help share the message that food is medicine.

Contents

CONTENTS

part four | RECIPES

Introduction

I was twenty-four years old, in school training to become a doctor of functional medicine and working as a clinical nutritionist just outside of Orlando, Florida, when I received a phone call from home. My mother, Winona, was on the line, and she sounded upset.

"What's wrong, Mom?" I asked.

"The cancer has come back," she said through tears.

My heart sank, and I was immediately transported back to my seventh-grade year, when my mom was told that she had stage 4 breast cancer that had spread to her lymph nodes. The news was not only a devastating blow to me, as her son—but it was also a shock to anyone who knew her. At the time, my mom was forty-one years old; she was my gym teacher at school and a swim instructor. Everyone thought she was the picture of fitness and health.

Soon after her diagnosis, my mom underwent a total mastectomy of her left breast and started the first of what would be four cycles of chemotherapy that left her too weak to get out of bed in the days that followed. It was painful to see how sick she got on chemo. I remember walking into the bathroom one day and seeing clumps of her sandy-blond hair on the floor. She looked like she had aged twenty years in two weeks.

Thankfully, months later she was declared cancer-free, but her health continued to spiral downward. Even after bouncing back from chemotherapy and returning to her job, she felt lousy. Every day, she would get home at three thirty in the afternoon and nap until dinner-time. We'd eat together but she struggled to stay awake and would turn in for the night soon after. When she told her doctor that she couldn't cope with being a wife, mother, and schoolteacher, he prescribed an antidepressant.

Depressed and exhausted: this was the mother I knew throughout my teenage years. She lived in fear that the cancer would return.

And now, ten years later, it had.

Her distressed voice shook me back to the present. "My oncologist told me they found a tumor on my lungs that was 2.5 centimeters," she said. "He wants to do surgery and start radiation and chemotherapy right away."

I tried to be as encouraging as possible. "Mom, please don't worry. Your body has the ability to heal," I said. "We just need to stop feeding the cancer cells and get to the root cause of the disease." I was confident her health could be restored—but, in order to do that, we'd need to take care of her whole body.

The next day, I flew home to help her lay out a health program. I asked her to tell me about any symptoms she had been experiencing in the time leading up to her diagnosis.

She sighed. "Well, I'm still struggling with depression," she said. "And even if I get a good night's sleep, I'm always tired the next day." She described symptoms that indicated she had multiple food sensitivities. She also revealed that she'd been diagnosed with hypothyroidism.

All of this was quite troubling—but it was her last symptom that shocked me. When I asked about her digestive habits, she revealed that she'd had an average of one to two bowel movements a week, for the last ten years.

"Wow, Mom," I said, stunned. "Why didn't you talk to your doctor about this earlier?"

"I thought it was normal," she said. Her face crumpled.

I reached out for her hand and told her not to be discouraged. "Mom," I said, "this is actually *good* news. We can definitely do some-thing about your digestion, and that alone will make a big difference in how you're feeling." *And hopefully will help stop the cancer, too*, I thought.

I told my mother about leaky gut syndrome—a condition in which the intestinal wall breaks down, allowing microbes and food particles to leak out of the digestive tract, triggering an inflammatory immune response—and how dangerous it was. I told her I believed it was the cause of her constipation and several other health problems, and that we needed to address it immediately. "We can do this, Mom," I said. "Come on." I stood up and asked her to follow me into the kitchen.

I grabbed a black garbage bag and opened kitchen cupboards. "We're starting all over," I announced. "From now on, you're not eating anything that comes out of a box."

Together, we threw out every processed food we could find:

- boxed cereals like Honey Nut Cheerios and Honey Bunches of Oats (she thought these cereals were healthy)
- plastic bottles of Juicy Juice billed as "90 percent real fruit juice" but made with apple juice concentrate and "natural" flavors that weren't natural at all
- chips and crackers made with MSG and genetically modified corn
- cereal bars made with high fructose corn syrup, artificial colors, and soy protein
- salad dressings with artificial thickeners, emulsifiers, and hydrogenated oils
- bags of highly refined white sugar and white flour

Then we attacked the refrigerator and tossed out condiments, sauces, margarine, coffee creamers, mayonnaise, and conventional dairy items such as skim milk and processed cheese ("American cheese") singles. Altogether, we threw out three huge garbage bags of processed foods.

Then we drove to a local health food store, where I walked her through the aisles and talked her through the types of foods she should be eating to help support her body in its fight to kill the cancer cells. We selected organic vegetables and berries, wild-caught salmon, pasture-raised chicken, and "clean" pantry staples—all organic foods with as few ingredients and as little processing as possible. Then we drove to another health food store, where we picked up nutritional supplements like turmeric, immune-boosting mushrooms, vitamin D$_3$, and frankincense essential oil.

At that time, the mainstream antibacterial craze was at its height, and almost every product in conventional grocery stores—from floor cleaner to toothpaste to number-two pencils—seemed to have added antibacterial ingredients. Scientists had started to sound the alarm about the overprescription of antibiotics causing resistance to some strains of illnesses, and the danger of overly sterile environments to our immune systems, but their research wasn't trickling down to most neighborhoods just yet. The evidence of these issues was showing up every day in my natural medicine practice, though. For several years I had seen the collateral damage these antibacterials and other supposedly "sanitary" chemicals were causing.

If part of the problem centered on being too clean, I felt certain the solution must be the opposite—to get dirty. To consciously create repeated "microexposures" to dirt that held long-lost bacteria, viruses, and other microbes that could function as nature's immunizations. To fortify and replenish the beneficial bacteria our bodies lost during the onslaught of antibacterial products in our environment. To completely reeducate the immune system, so it could once again learn how to defend itself without going overboard.

To not be afraid of a little dirt here and there, but instead, more consciously follow the rhythms of nature and embrace the healing power that surrounds us every day.

And so, to start Mom's healing program, I went straight for the dirt. In my years of medical research, I'd developed a special interest in probiotics—supplements and foods rich in healthy microorganisms, bacteria, fungi, and yeast that tip the overall balance of our gut microbiota toward health. One of the most novel and interesting threads of research I'd found centered on microorganisms in soil, which possesses many vital microbes often missing in the human body. Right away, I started my mom on a probiotic supplement with soil-based organisms (SBOs) believed to improve the absorption of nutrients, eliminate yeast overgrowth, and improve bowel function.

Then I brainstormed other ways for my mom to "get dirty." She liked to ride horses growing up, so she headed back to the stables and began riding regularly, breathing in dust and grooming the horses. We also visited the farmer's market to pick up organic, locally grown produce that had traveled less than ten miles from the farm. The vegetables were vibrant with antioxidants and had clumps of soil still clinging to their roots. In her kitchen, I taught my mom how to make green drinks with servings of spinach, celery, cucumber, cilantro, lime, green apple, and stevia. She consumed a daily regimen of supplements, high-quality extracts derived from medicinal plants. She downed many cups of bone broth soup, the healing elixir made from the bones and innards of chicken, beef, lamb, or fish—animal parts previously considered dirty waste, now known to be an excellent source of collagen, glutamine, and other nutrients that help "heal and seal" the lining of the gut. She spent time outside in her garden every day, digging in the flower beds, or simply being still and giving thanks.

I have to hand it to Mom—she followed my diet and lifestyle advice very closely. And over the next several months, she saw many positive changes in her health: her constipation problems resolved, and she began having one bowel movement every day. She noticed a major upswing in her energy. Her thyroid issues disappeared. She lost twenty-two pounds, and she no longer felt depressed. She reported feeling more joy than she had ever experienced.

When my mom went in four months later for a CT scan, her surgeons were mystified by the results. Not only was her blood work normal, her cancer markers had dropped dramatically.

"What's happened is very unusual," the oncologist said, with obvious surprise. "We don't see cancer shrink very often." Her largest tumor had shrunk by 52 percent.

The oncologist encouraged her to keep doing what she was doing, "because whatever it is, it's working." Her medical team decided to hold off on surgery. Mom was greatly relieved to avoid going under the knife again.

Now, I want to be clear: cancer is one of the most extreme health concerns any of us will ever face. I would never claim that my program "cured" my mom's cancer. Many factors come into play with an outcome like hers, and she was very diligent about following the guidance and directions of her other doctors. But where her doctors' instructions left off, her diet and lifestyle changes began. And I believe it is due to the integration of all of these factors that today—more than twenty years after she first learned she had breast cancer, and a decade after this second diagnosis—Mom is enjoying the fruits of her lifestyle changes.

About seven years after her second diagnosis, my mom and dad retired and moved to a house on a lake in Florida. Today, they enjoy water-skiing and hiking trails with new friends. Mom has run several 5K races with me (finishing in second and third place in her age group!). She is radiant and bursting with energy. Almost every time I see her, she marvels at how much her health has changed. She says she feels better in her sixties than she did in her thirties!

BONUS: If you want the detailed eating plan, supplement plan, and lifestyle regimen my mom followed to heal herself, you can download it for free at: www.draxe.com/healing-plan-bonus

---

I can't tell you how grateful I feel for my mother's health—she is and will always be my greatest inspiration. Those awful months of pain and agony she endured when she was first diagnosed with breast cancer were what made me decide to become a doctor. And the experience of helping her heal her leaky gut—and subsequently overcome her hypothyroidism, chronic fatigue, depression, and cancer—crystallized my life's mission as a medical professional. To me, her vibrant health makeover perfectly epitomizes the power of full-body healing that can take place when you first heal your gut.

The protocol that she followed, the same approach I've used with thousands of patients, forms the backbone of the Eat Dirt program. I believe this approach holds tremendous promise for revolutionizing our nation's health—and not a moment too soon. We are experiencing a hidden epidemic of leaky gut.

— A Kick to the Gut —

While the term "leaky gut" still draws skepticism and smirks from some in the media and medical community, its more precise medical term—

"increased intestinal permeability"—has been thoroughly documented in the medical literature for over a hundred years, and more recently as a recognized risk factor for autoimmune disease. The prevalence of this devastating condition is clearly rising, as witnessed by a parallel upsurge in autoimmune disease in the past decade. The worldwide prevalence for type 1 diabetes, a condition with proven links to leaky gut, rose almost 40 percent between 1998 and 2008 alone.[1] Today, an estimated 50 million Americans—almost one in six—struggle with autoimmune conditions. The total number of autoimmune conditions now approaches one hundred, with an additional forty conditions suspected of having an autoimmune basis.[2] And while researchers are still working on articulating the exact mechanisms involved, functional medicine clinicians have found that many disparate conditions—including allergies, asthma, food sensitivities, digestive diseases, arthritis, thyroid conditions, even frustratingly difficult-to-treat conditions such as chronic fatigue and autism—either greatly improve or completely resolve with the introduction and judicious application of a leaky gut protocol.

Our nation is in the grip of a hidden epidemic. We've been taking our digestive system for granted for far too long, starving it of actual nutrition while overfeeding it with toxic levels of processed foods and sugar and overtaxing it with environmental chemicals, stress, and excessive antimicrobials. We've long viewed the digestive system merely as being responsible for converting food into energy, or helping to regulate metabolism, or ridding the body of waste products. Clearly this view has been woefully incomplete, and has obstructed the essential truth: the gut is not simply a food-processing center—the gut is the center of health itself.

— Sealing Up Our Defenses —

The signs of leaky gut can be confusingly varied:

You might feel tired and sluggish.
You could get frequent indigestion, heartburn, bloating, and gas.
You might develop sensitivities to certain foods, foods that
    you've enjoyed without incident for years (or decades).

You can experience persistent "brain fog," characterized by a cloudy memory and lack of focus.

You may notice changes in your skin, such as dark circles under your eyes, or inflamed skin conditions such as eczema, psoriasis, and acne.

If the situation persists, you might start to develop more serious ramifications: chronic fatigue, adrenal exhaustion, and lethargy. Crippling pain and arthritis. A range of dangerous digestive conditions, including inflammatory bowel disease. Autoimmune diseases like Hashimoto's thyroiditis. Sometimes, frighteningly, inexplicably life-threatening conditions.

If you had never heard about leaky gut and didn't know the connections, you might spend years chasing down each symptom or condition, seeking relief from your allergist, cardiologist, rheumatologist, endocrinologist, neurologist—or even psychologist. All these disparate symptoms, with just one source? Could the answer be that simple? And if the prevalence of these conditions is rising so quickly and dramatically, how on earth can we protect ourselves?

Thankfully, the answer is in our hands—and in our kitchens, farms, backyards, subways, and schools.

We need to *eat dirt*.

— The Eat Dirt Solution —

While the effects of leaky gut can be devastating, the solutions are simple, affordable, and widely available, all fully within the grasp of every person reading these words.

In this book, I'll share everything I've learned about leaky gut and how to heal from it. We'll talk about how leaky gut syndrome begins and the trajectory of its development. We'll dig deep into the risk factors of this condition, and why it has become a major cause of disease and dysfunction in our country and around the world. We'll talk about how you can determine if you have leaky gut, and how you can protect yourself and your family—starting today.

Together, using the tools in this book, we'll develop a personalized protocol that can begin to heal and seal your gut, tamp down inflammation, reduce immune dysfunction, and radically improve your health, both in your immediate future and over your entire lifespan. After implementing the strategies outlined in this book, not only will you greatly reduce your risk of disease, you'll also notice changes such as:

- ▶ improved energy
- ▶ restored digestion
- ▶ glowing, healthy-looking skin
- ▶ clear sinuses and fewer allergic symptoms
- ▶ pain-free joints
- ▶ mental clarity and focus
- ▶ improved body image and confidence
- ▶ increased metabolism (and fewer pounds)
- ▶ hormone balance
- ▶ fewer emotional ups and downs

In part 1, we'll begin by describing the hidden epidemic that is leaky gut. We'll talk about the signs and symptoms of leaky gut, how it starts and progresses, and how it is believed to be the root of some of the most common yet devastating health conditions. (Take the quiz at the end of chapter 1 to gauge your own risk for leaky gut.) We'll talk about our vast, mysterious universe within—the trillions of bacterial cells that make up our microbiome—and how we've only just begun to understand the scope of its role in our physical and mental health. We'll talk about how we have endangered our beneficial bacteria through many of our lifestyle excesses and environmental toxins, connecting the dots between leaky gut and our growing epidemic of autoimmune conditions. And we'll end part 1 with a discussion of the most promising solution: turning the clock back on many of our sanitizing, antibacterial, overly "clean" modern habits. By returning to some of the simple practices of everyday life, we can actually protect our beneficial bacteria and strengthen our immune systems. We'll talk about how many ancient practices that seemed the least sterile actually kept us strong for millennia. We'll also discuss how the advent of modern conveniences—refrigeration, industrial agriculture, daily showers—as well as rampant antibiotics and other weapons in our ill-advised war on germs left us more vulnerable. Finally, we'll talk about how "dirt"—both metaphorical and literal—has the power to rebuild the gut barrier. Our gut lining is the front line of our immune system. When we care for it well, it can help nourish us by allowing in the right balance of micronutrients while remaining tough as nails against our pathogenic foes.

In part 2, we'll go through five major modern "improvements" intended to protect humans from harm that instead backfired completely, leaving us vulnerable to many of the same diseases and maladies we initially sought to prevent. We'll discuss how the modern food supply, environmental toxins, excessive stress, oversanitation, and pharmaceutical medicines all increased the toxic load in the body, leaving it overwhelmed and defenseless against true threats, including antibiotic-resistant microbes, deadly viruses, genuine allergens, and our own preexisting genetic risks. We'll talk about simple, pleasurable changes we can make in our daily lives to address and reverse each of these critical missteps. These changes not only heal leaky gut and improve our health but can enrich and deepen our connection to the natural world. The Eat Dirt philosophy helps bring a healthy rhythm back into our lives, and ultimately creates a more sustainable planet for our children.

Then, we will put all the pieces together into the Eat Dirt lifestyle program, a five-step plan to help remove the toxins in your gut, replenish and fortify the beneficial balance of your microbiota, and restore your healthy gut lining so your entire body can thrive.

Once you've implemented the core program, in part 3, you can further refine it to address your unique profile by taking an online quiz to determine which of the five most common gut types best describes your individual issues or lingering concerns. Based on specific personal health and lifestyle risk factors, I'll suggest targeted strategies that boost the effectiveness of the core program for each of these five gut types:

- ▶ **Candida gut,** directly related to yeast overgrowth and being overweight, which affects more than 68 percent of all American adults.[3]
- ▶ **Stressed gut,** in which chronic stress weakens your adrenal glands, kidneys, and thyroid, and can cause hormone imbalances, fatigue, and thyroid disease.

▶ **Immune gut,** which afflicts the 15 million people who suffer from food allergies[4] and the 1.6 million with inflammatory bowel disease,[5] as well as the 50 million adults with autoimmune disease.[6]

▶ **Gastric gut,** caused by small intestinal bacteria overgrowth (SIBO) and acid reflux, which afflicts 60 percent of all adults—half of whom struggle on a weekly basis.

▶ **Toxic gut,** which can result in gallbladder disease, skin conditions, and chronic liver issues that cause thirty million people great pain every year.[7]

For each of these gut types, I share customized recommendations and offer specific advice about which foods to eat or avoid, what nutritional supplements best meet your needs, and what additional steps you might take to optimize your transformation to a healthy gut. (We'll also discuss how to modify the program if you suspect that you may have a hybrid gut type.)

To help make implementing the Eat Dirt program as easy as possible, I've included dozens of my patients' favorite healthy recipes for meals, as well as guidelines to create personal care and cleaning products that replace toxic chemicals with healing essential oils. The Eat Dirt resource guide at the end of the book will help you locate healing foods and supplements, farmer's markets, and other resources in your community or online. Along the way, I'll share stories of many of my patients to illustrate how this simple approach—to return to the "dirty" practices that once supported and strengthened our immune system—has the power to remedy many long-standing health issues, and return you to your natural state of radiant health.

— Time to Get Dirty —

The Eat Dirt program has evolved over my many years in practice. I've tested these treatments on thousands of patients and have observed firsthand the transformative effects they experience once their gut health has been restored. For more than a decade, I've followed the medical journals, watching as scientific validation has accumulated, documenting the phenomena I've witnessed daily both clinically and in my own personal life. I'll present some of that research here, the findings of which very clearly point to the fact that our guts are hurting and need our help.

I have faith that if you follow the guidelines in this book, you will experience an amazing improvement in your overall health—not just better digestion, but more energy, weight loss, better mood, and so much more. I hope that once you do, you will join me in spreading the word about leaky gut, and teach your family and your neighbors how they, too, can tap the power of dirt to reverse their immune system challenges.

We are all part of an enormous ecosystem that's in need of healing—and one by one, we can be a part of the solution. Time to dig in and get dirty. The health of the planet rests in our hands—and our guts!

— part one —

WHY WE'RE SUFFERING

1

The Hidden Epidemic

All disease begins in the gut.
—HIPPOCRATES, THE FATHER OF MEDICINE

Miriam walked into my office almost out of hope. She'd run the gamut from conventional family doctors to holistic physicians and, despite following her doctors' varied directions, had experienced minimal improvement. I was the *tenth* health professional she'd consulted in her quest to turn her health around.

At thirty-three years old with two young children, Miriam was twenty pounds overweight—and 100 percent stressed out. She'd been diagnosed with Hashimoto's thyroiditis, a disease in which the immune system attacks the thyroid, and was prescribed the medication Synthroid by her endocrinologist. She'd also taken antianxiety medications and antidepressants, but they hadn't helped. Her mental and emotional stress had caused a naturopathic physician to diagnose adrenal fatigue, and blood tests revealed a deficiency in vitamin B_{12}. She'd tried to change her diet and had even been receiving vitamin B_{12} shots once a week for the last two years—but nothing was working. She wanted to exercise, but she could barely summon the energy to get out of bed in the morning. And like many young mothers, once the kids were awake, she had very little time for fitness classes or working out.

Miriam was sick of feeling tired all the time—something had to change.

When I reviewed her three-day food diary, I could see that Miriam was eating a surprisingly good diet. She ate quite a few salads, slices of sprouted grain bread, plenty of fruits and vegetables—but the nutrient content of her food just didn't seem to be helping.

I ordered a blood test so I could double-check her previous results. When I got them back, it was clear that, indeed, nothing had changed. Her descriptions of thyroid problems, adrenal fatigue, autoimmune disease, and food sensitivities were all reflected in the numbers.

Miriam came in the next week so we could review the report together. With each set of numbers, she looked more and more dejected. Wanting to reassure her, I set down the lab results and reached for two of my favorite props that I kept handy in my examination room: a small fishing net and a handful of brightly colored plastic balls.

"Ready?" She nodded. "Check this out." I dropped the plastic balls into the fishing net. Miriam, expecting them to be caught by the net, gasped and looked startled as they fell through the bottom and bounced all over the wooden floor.

"Didn't expect that, huh?" I said. She shook her head.

"Miriam," I said, "I'm afraid that net is your gut."

I showed her how the strings at the bottom of the net had been severed, to illustrate what happens in leaky gut syndrome. When our guts are healthy, I explained, the intestines are only slightly permeable, like the thin mesh of an intact net, to allow minute quantities of water and nutrients through the gut's thin barrier and into the bloodstream—a normal, necessary part of digestion, and an essential step in nourishing the body.

"However, when the holes in the intestinal wall get too big, larger molecules, such as gluten and casein, and other foreign microbes can pass through and start wandering all over the body," I explained, gesturing to the balls still rolling around the examining room floor. These larger items were never meant to hit the bloodstream, I said, and the body reacts to them as foreign bodies, causing systemic inflammation throughout the body.

Any organ in the body can be affected when this happens. "In your case, it's your thyroid, brain, and adrenal glands," I said.

I told Miriam that no matter how many vitamin B shots she received or how many supplements she took, if she didn't fix the root cause of the problem—her leaky gut—she would continue to face all the same, ever-mounting challenges. But now that we knew about the problem, I felt confident she could see significant improvements in a short time. All she needed to do was follow my recommendations and make just a few changes to her diet and daily habits.

I gave Miriam a healing protocol that started with foods high in probiotics—good bacteria that could tame her digestive problems—and prebiotics—foods with compatible nutrients that would feed those good bacteria. I asked her to make a smoothie using kefir and flaxseeds as the main ingredients to start off the morning, and to drink multiple cups of bone broth throughout the day, to help seal the lining of her gut. To help reduce her stress hormones, I urged her to find time for two or three fifteen-minute walks through the neighborhood and to take a healing bath with Epsom salts and lavender essential oil every night.

After two weeks, Miriam came back for a follow-up. In that brief time, she'd lost five pounds and noticed that she had considerably more energy. Encouraged, she pledged to follow her health plan for ninety days, at which point we would redo her blood work.

Three months later, the results spoke for themselves.

In just three months, Miriam's vitamin B_{12} deficiency had reverted to normal levels. Her cortisol levels had dropped, as had her triglycerides, fasting blood sugar and insulin, and CRP, a marker of systemic inflammation. Best of all, when her endocrinologist received her lab test results, he called to congratulate her on her progress and announce that he wanted to reduce her Synthroid dosage by 75 percent.

When she came into my office to review her results in person, Miriam's face looked rosy and her eyes sparkled. "I can't believe how much energy I have," she gushed, smiling as she took her shoes off and hopped onto the scale. "I can finally run around with the boys again!" Then her eyes widened as she saw the readout on the scale: she'd lost twenty-seven pounds since her first appointment.

I have treated many hundreds of Miriams over the years. Her case is a perfect example of how sneaky leaky gut can be, how well it disguises itself as other conditions, how progressive and cumulative its effects can be—and yet how incredibly effective a few very simple changes can be in helping to resolve it.

Having seen this exact scenario repeated thousands of times over my years in practice, I know there are many more thousands of people who are struggling as Miriam was when she first entered my office: sick and tired, and rapidly losing hope. I firmly believe that the only things that are holding us back from reversing our country's affliction of leaky gut are awareness, knowledge, and faith—both about the existence of leaky gut and our ability to solve it.

We *can* heal. We just need to summon the collective will to change some of our long-standing but extremely damaging habits—especially our deadly addiction to being clean.

— The Serious Condition with the Silly Name —

I'm going to guess that the first time you heard the phrase "leaky gut," you thought it was a joke. *Do you honestly expect me to believe my stomach has sprung a leak?* I understand that the name itself may be a bit of stumbling block for some. But once people get past the distraction of the silly name, they start to see how virulent, widespread, and devastating this hidden epidemic has become.

With a surface area of about 200 square meters—about the size of a tennis court—our digestive tract is a vital immune barrier, protecting us from disease and contamination. Every day, thousands of microorganisms and by-products of digestion come into contact with this critical defense shield. This clever gut lining has a tricky job to do: distinguishing the contents of the intestines from the body's own tissues, managing the absorption of nutrients, and generally overseeing the interaction between the resident microbial population and the mucosal immune system. In fact, between these activities and killing foreign invaders, the gut lining accounts for 70 percent of our immune system.[1]

To keep us in good health, our gut relies on carefully maintaining a symbiotic relationship with trillions of microorganisms, the cells of which outnumber our human cells by a factor of ten to one.[2] These microorganisms are a mix of good guys (mutualists), bad guys (pathogens), and neutral bystanders (commensals) that basically just go with the flow.[3] Most experts believe the average healthy mix of microbes is about 85 percent positive/neutral and 15 percent negative, which creates a lively balance that keeps the immune system well trained and on its toes to defend against unhealthy viruses and other antigens.[4]

Every time we ingest something, the immune system in our gut must discern what is friend and what is foe, either welcoming or expelling nutrients, microorganisms, bacteria, and bugs. A healthy immune system remains quietly vigilant, like a burly bouncer, admitting the good and swiftly dispatching the bad. But when the gut gets mobbed by a relentless, unruly crowd—toxins in the environment, a nutrient-deficient diet, stress, medications, or other factors—the bouncer gets overwhelmed and our defenses are weakened. That's when opportunistic bad bacteria make their move. These troublemakers take advantage of our impaired immunity and find their way in.

Once they have their foothold, those bad bacteria can change the environment in the gut. They crowd out the good bacterial citizens that make their home there, take the place of probiotics that are responsible for vitamin production, burrow into mucus on the gut wall, and create holes in the intestinal lining that can change the pH balance of the gut and lead to yeast overgrowth. As a result, the outermost layer of the gut barrier, the epithelium, starts to weaken. The junctions between its cells normally function as tightly controlled gates, preventing unwanted molecules from seeping into the bloodstream. But when the gut wall is weakened, these gates can open up and stay open much longer than anyone would want, allowing toxins, microbes, and undigested food particles to leak directly into the bloodstream and travel throughout the body.

Now, all of us experience leaky gut at one point or another, but we might never know it. When those microbes sneak out, our immune system releases antibodies that neutralize the invaders, and that's that. But when leaky gut becomes chronic, the toxic potential of those roaming microbes means leaky gut is no longer a localized, fleeting digestive issue—it becomes a systemic syndrome that can have significant, widespread, and even deadly health ramifications. The body's inflammatory response—a result of your immune system trying to protect you—can get locked in the "on" position, and start attacking everything and any-

How Leaky Gut Develops

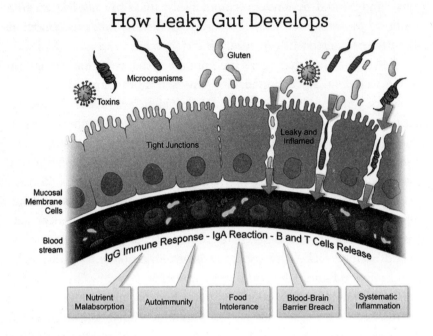

thing in its path. When this happens, you become at risk of developing a lifelong, debilitating autoimmune condition.

So yes, leaky gut may be a silly name. But as I hope you're beginning to see, it is most definitely a serious condition than can wreak havoc on your health.

— A Serious Condition That's Becoming More Prevalent —

Upon their initial visit, approximately 80 percent of my patients present with some level of leaky gut syndrome. They come to my clinic experiencing problems ranging from gallbladder issues to thyroid disease, psoriasis or eczema, migraine headaches, insulin resistance, and even stubborn weight gain. Many are amazed to learn that their condition may share the same origin as colitis, irritable bowel syndrome (IBS), and Crohn's disease. And they're downright stunned when I tell them that some degree of leaky gut is present in every autoimmune disease, including lupus, multiple sclerosis (MS), type 1 diabetes, and even

Parkinson's and ALS. What I try not to mention is that they might have started down the same road to some of those more serious conditions had they not come to me when they did.

Many mainstream medical groups eschew the term "leaky gut syndrome," preferring the more technically specific term "increased intestinal permeability." But that difference in terminology is quickly becoming irrelevant, as the field explodes with new information about our gut's (and our microbiome's) impact on human health and behavior. Health professionals and researchers from all disciplines are coming together to share information, and the field is advancing daily, with more than twelve hundred studies on intestinal permeability published in the last year alone. All this research is helping to connect the dots and confirm what naturopathic doctors, integrative specialists, and other experts in functional medicine have been sounding the alarm about for years: our modern environmental toxic load is too vast, our food is too nutritionally bankrupt, and our lives are too stressful for our bodies to thrive. The intestine's microbial balance and extremely delicate gut lining can only take so much abuse before the barrier breaks down and the bad guys start to get through. And once that happens, all bets are off.

According to research conducted on both animal and human subjects and published in journals such as *Clinical Gastroenterology and Hepatology* and *Gut*,[5] leaky gut syndrome (or increased intestinal permeability) has been linked to the following symptoms and conditions:

ALS (Lou Gehrig's disease)[6]
Alzheimer's disease[7]
Anxiety and depression[8]
ADHD (attention deficit hyperactivity disorder)[9]
Autism[10]
Candida and yeast overgrowth[11]
Celiac disease and nonceliac gluten sensitivity[12]
Chronic fatigue syndrome[13]
Crohn's disease[14]
Fibromyalgia[15]
Gas, bloating, and digestive pain[16]
Hashimoto's disease[17]
Irritable bowel syndrome[18]

Lupus[19]

Metabolic syndrome[20]

Migraine headaches[21]

Multiple sclerosis[22]

NAFLD (nonalcoholic fatty liver disease) and other liver
  malfunction[23]

Parkinson's disease[24]

PCOS (polycystic ovarian syndrome)[25]

Restless leg syndrome[26]

Rheumatoid arthritis[27]

Skin inflammation (eczema, psoriasis, rosacea, dermatitis, and
  acne)[28]

Type 1 diabetes[29, 30]

Type 2 diabetes[31]

Ulcerative colitis[32]

Various allergies and food sensitivities[33]

And this list is by no means comprehensive. The research on leaky
gut is growing rapidly—who knows what we will discover in the next
ten years?

The links are so strong, and the evidence so compelling, we can no
longer pretend this is just a fad condition with a silly name. Leaky gut is
at ground zero of many of the country's most confounding health crises.

— But Why Is This Happening? —

So why now? What is happening in our world to create this hidden epidemic? While any one factor could cause problems for our guts, several
of these are converging at once, creating a perfect storm in the gut.

The corruption of the food supply. The unrelenting surplus of excess
sugars; unsprouted, hybridized grains; and other nutritionally bankrupt,
processed foods has simply devastated the gut. Of particular concern
is gluten, which evidence increasingly points to as a prime driver of
leaky gut. When it's consumed, the body undergoes an inflammatory
response and eventually releases the protein—zonulin—that unlocks

the epithelial tight junctions and keeps the gates of the gut wide open as long as it circulates in the blood.[34]

The rise of environmental toxins. Each of us has the potential to come into contact with as many as eighty thousand untested environmental chemicals and toxins over the course of a single year. Our country represents less than 2 percent of the world's population, but we use 24 percent of its pesticides.[35] The widespread use of these pesticides, combined with the presence in our lives and diets of genetically modified crops, food additives and preservatives, and even household cleaners and beauty products, has created a dangerous toxic load in our bodies that has degraded our gut health.

The overwhelming stress of modern life. Emotional stress exacts a very real toll on our gut health. Research has shown that stressful life experiences cause a decrease in probiotic diversity, which allows overgrowth of yeast in the gut. Stress also weakens the immune system over time, crippling our ability to fight off foreign invaders like bad bacteria and viruses, exacerbating any preexisting inflammation, and perpetuating leaky gut.

Unrelenting germ warfare. Our culture's addiction to oversanitizing our hands and our homes, treating every ailment under the sun with broad-spectrum antibiotics, and overprocessing our food has corrupted our innate microbial balance. We've killed off many strains of beneficial microbes that used to fine-tune our genes and strategically train our immune systems to handle pathogens, allergens, and other threatening factors in the environment. This disruption of our gut's healthy coexistence with the phytobiome, nature's vast universe of microbes, has had deadly consequences, including a rise in related chronic disease, autoimmune dysfunction, and antibiotic resistance. This year, at least two million people will become infected with antibiotic-resistant bacteria, and twenty-three thousand people will die as a result.[36]

Overuse of medication. With seven in ten Americans on at least one prescription medication, NSAIDs and other painkillers consumed at record levels, and antibiotics readily prescribed, synthetic drugs have hurt our guts by compromising our mucosal barrier, damaging our intestinal villi, and killing off beneficial bacteria on an unfathomable scale. One Stanford University study found that a single course of ciprofloxacin antibiotics could wipe out 50 percent of a baby's gut microbiome in as little as four days. And while most of the bacteria bounced back, in some children certain individual strains never rebounded, and were lost for good.[37]

While any one of these factors could increase our risk of developing leaky gut, most of us face several. Think back to the story of my mom: she'd eaten the standard American diet all her life, received an antibiotic prescription any time she'd felt a bug coming on, and faced extraordinary emotional difficulties since she was a child. She developed ulcers and food allergies at an early age, and when she was just eleven years old, had been diagnosed with gastritis, an inflammation and irritation of the lining of the stomach. She grew up thinking that stomachaches and infrequent bowel movements were normal. But the reason she'd had so many seemingly unrelated health issues and had felt so poorly for most of her life—long before cancer struck—was leaky gut, most likely developed during childhood.

Almost all of us have swallowed ibuprofen for a headache, eaten processed foods, washed our hands with antibacterial soap, taken an antibiotic, or experienced chronic stress. Any of these on its own could damage the gut; combine a few of them, and leaky gut becomes almost inevitable. And just like a boat that's sprung a leak, no amount of bailing will keep our overall health afloat if we don't first stop to fix the leak.

— The Solution Is Simple —

As we've moved from agrarian to industrial to urban/suburban life, we've slowly distanced ourselves from many of the things that make us who we are. On a cell-for-cell basis, we are 90 percent microbial. We don't just live on the earth—the earth lives in us. In order for our inner and outer ecosystems to peacefully coexist and support one another, we need to combine the best of modern life with those simple practices that kept us healthy and disease-free for many years.

We need to start seeing those countless strains of bacteria, viruses, phages, parasites, and other microbes as old friends that we're welcoming back into our guts, so they can start protecting us again. This "old friends" theory holds that if we can reclaim our microbial diversity through microexposures—small, repeated exposures to the "dirt," such as bacteria, soil, dust, plant oils—we can reestablish the natural symbiotic relationship that we've always had with these microbes. Like nature's immunizations, these microexposures keep a steady stream of good bugs coming into our system, interacting with our genes, and strengthening our immune system by reinforcing and teaching our native gut colonies how best to interact with the world around us.

While this is cutting-edge science, the solutions could not be any simpler. All we need to do to load up on our old friends and get more of these microexposures is easy, fun stuff we probably already love to do: Get back to eating seasonally and locally. Spend more time outdoors. Hug our dogs after they roll around in the leaves. Let our kids make mud pies and get their hands dirty on the playground.

And to make sure our old friends feel safe and stick around, there are also a few things that we shouldn't do: Freak out about germs. Blast everything with sanitizers. Take a pill for every single ache or pain.

Simply put: we need to *eat dirt*. We can reverse many of our missteps, heal our gut, and recover from many of these diseases by making more basic and bacteria-rich choices in what we eat and how we live. And just by living that simpler way of life, with all of those daily microexposures to nature in all its dirty, microbial bounty, we will finally be able to repopulate the gut with those old friends that bring balance and help restore our radiant health.

We will get into all the specifics of exactly how we can do that in parts 2 and 3. But first, let's take a closer look at exactly what leaky gut is and how it happens, so we'll know exactly what we need to do about it, in every area of our lives.

— Do You Have Leaky Gut? —

At this point in our discussion, you may be wondering if you have leaky gut—or you may be starting to realize that there is a real term for the varied symptoms you've been experiencing for years. I estimate that eight out of every ten of my patients have some degree of leaky gut. You may be very low on the inflammation scale, with just a few symptoms such as bloating or fatigue. Or you may be experiencing chronic inflammation, with several severe symptoms that interfere with your daily life. Just as with most diseases, there is a spectrum of severity when it comes to leaky gut. Answer the questions below to get a sense of your risk and where you fall on the scale.

LEAKY GUT QUIZ

BONUS: To take the full-color version of the quiz with recommendations from Dr. Axe go to www.draxe.com/leaky-gut-quiz

1. Are you currently taking any prescription medications or over-the-counter drugs like aspirin or ibuprofen?
   ☐ yes   ☐ no

2. Do you have thyroid issues or sluggish metabolism?
   ☐ yes   ☐ no

3. Do you have low energy or frequent fatigue?
   ☐ yes   ☐ no

4. Do you have frequent diarrhea or loose stools?
   ☐ yes   ☐ no

5. Do you have gas, bloating, or any other digestive issues once or more per week?
   ☐ yes   ☐ no

6. Have you been diagnosed with an autoimmune disease?
☐ yes   ☐ no

7. Do you struggle with seasonal allergies?
☐ yes   ☐ no

8. Are your bowel movements soft on a regular basis?
☐ yes   ☐ no

9. Do you get sick often, meaning two or more times a year, and do you feel like you need an immune system boost?
☐ yes   ☐ no

10. Do you ever go more than one day without a bowel movement?
☐ yes   ☐ no

11. Are your stress levels moderate to high?
☐ yes   ☐ no

12. Do you have skin conditions like rosacea, eczema, acne, or rashes?
☐ yes   ☐ no

13. Do you crave sweets or breads?
☐ yes   ☐ no

14. Do you struggle with depression, anxiety, or lack of focus?
☐ yes   ☐ no

15. Have you ever struggled with any type of candida, yeast, or fungal issues, or do you have a white coating on your tongue?
☐ yes   ☐ no

16. Have you been diagnosed with ulcerative colitis, Crohn's disease, or IBS?
☐ yes   ☐ no

17. Do you suffer from any type of pain, including joint pain or head-aches?

☐ yes   ☐ no

18. Are you sensitive to gluten or dairy?

☐ yes   ☐ no

19. Do you have an autoimmune disease like Hashimoto's thyroiditis, psoriasis, or multiple sclerosis?

☐ yes   ☐ no

20. Do you have multiple food sensitivities or food allergies (such as gluten or dairy)?

☐ yes   ☐ no

If you answered yes to fewer than two questions, you are currently very low on the leaky gut scale; with proper care, your gut should remain strong.

If you answered yes to two or three questions, you may have some low-level inflammatory response, and cleaning up your diet and changing your lifestyle will likely prevent you from developing full-blown leaky gut and autoimmune problems.

If you answered yes to more than four questions, there's a strong possibility that a prolonged case of leaky gut has already begun to manifest in more serious health issues. While you pursue treatment of your other symptoms, please also see the Gut Type Quiz preview (see page 186) to get more targeted relief as soon as possible.

Wherever you fall on the leaky gut spectrum, don't worry—you *can* heal your gut and reduce your inflammation. All you need to do is follow the Eat Dirt program and increase your microexposures to beneficial microbes in your daily life.

2

Ground Zero for Leaky Gut

These days, when people talk about the "gut," they're often referring to the trillions of residents that live inside the organs of our physical digestive system: the gut microbiome.

Our microbiome comprises all of the microorganisms (bacteria, viruses, fungi, yeast, parasites, and more) that reside in or on the human body. Although we are considered the "host" of these microbes, bacteria actually outnumber human cells by a factor of ten to one—with a hundred trillion in the intestines alone. (Think of that: *one hundred trillion*. You could spend a million dollars every single day since AD 1 and still not spend even $1 trillion by 2016.)

Experts estimate that if you could collect the microbes together living inside you (known as the microbiota), they'd weigh somewhere between two and six pounds—in other words, about twice the weight of the average human brain.[1]

Most of the microbiome lives inside your intestines, which is ground zero for where leaky gut takes place. The gut microbiota play an enormous role in many different biological functions, but perhaps their most important role is establishing and developing our immune system and protecting the integrity of the gut lining.

We have a symbiotic relationship with these tiny creatures: microbes depend on us as hosts, and the vast majority help to protect us from dangerous bacteria, regulate our metabolism, and aid in digestion. The bacteria work hard to digest food and create vitamins, manage our hormone levels, dispose of toxins, and create natural chemicals that help feed and protect the lining of the gut. A peaceful, mutually beneficial balance is maintained through many intersecting mechanisms, including gut secretions (for hormones, vitamins, and enzymes), movement of foods through the GI tract, the interactions of the bugs themselves, and more. If the microbes interact well with these processes (and each other), they protect the integrity of the gut lining, and with it, our immunity. When the balance is off, the fallout can be serious.

— Our Lifelong Companions —

Our microbial friends have known us for a long time. Even before birth, a baby is exposed to beneficial microbes (such as Firmicutes and Bacteroidetes) via the mother's placenta.[2] On the way out the mother's birth canal, that tiny baby boy or girl is exposed to trillions more, which lay the foundation for the microbiome—and the immune system—that baby will develop over the coming years. Pioneering doctors have even begun to dab babies born via C-sections with their mothers' vaginal secretions so they don't miss out on this foundational bacterial bath. With his or her first meal, another influx of microbes will arrive—because breast milk also contains microbes, including the very bacteria that help us to digest our mother's milk. What's amazing is that these bugs that we are exposed to in the very first hours of life are the seed starters of our microbiome and will help to determine the course of our gut health for the rest of our lives.

Now, if we continue to live our naturally dirty human lives—if we're breast-fed and live in a house with a dog and enjoy the time-honored baby activity of putting random things in our mouths—these microbiota will grow and thrive. Responding to the various microorganisms we encounter, we continue to pick up bugs here and there, adding to the general diversity in our gut. The number of species grows from about 100 when we're babies to about 1,000 when we're adults. The composition changes based on who's around, too, shifting from one that closely resembles Mom's to one that reflects both mom and dad, your brothers and sisters, or whoever cares for you as a baby.[3] But if we grow up in an extremely clean environment, without access to all that dirty goodness, we have fewer microexposures to both good and bad bugs, and our gut population will remain less diverse. And if we get sick somewhere along the way and need to be treated with an antibiotic (or several) during the first years of life, what diversity we have developed will be almost entirely wiped out—leaving the gut more vulnerable to virulent strains of bacteria, which can be incredibly crafty about survival.

— Diversity Will Save Us —

But it's not always the good guys that have the most numbers—sometimes dangerous pathogens are the ones that rule the microbiome. This overpopulation of bad guys is a common side effect of frequent antibiotic use. The Centers for Disease Control has issued threat alerts for new antibiotic-resistant bugs that infect more than two million people a year.[4] Four new antibiotic-resistant strains of salmonella have increased outbreaks in food-borne illnesses across the country.[5] Antibiotic-resistant *C. diff* infection is by far the most devastating, with its painful diarrhea, fever, and kidney failure. According to the CDC, we have almost five hundred thousand diagnoses per year, with twenty-nine thousand of these dying within thirty days of diagnosis.[6] Almost as many as die in car crashes[7] or from gunshot wounds.[8]

Terrifying, right? So how can we fight back?

Diversity.

Bacterial diversity keeps the whole system in balance.

A healthy gut contains so many different kinds of bugs that no one strain wins out. A highly respected study by a group of European scientists, published in the journal *Nature*, analyzed the microbiome of 229 people and separated them into two groups. People with fewer than 480,000 bacterial genes were termed "low gene count" (LGC) and the rest were considered "high gene count" (HGC). The richness of their microbiota differed by about 40 percent, and almost one in four of us would fall in the low gene count group. The researchers found this low level of bacterial richness corresponds with higher body weight and fat, insulin resistance, high cholesterol and triglycerides, and more pronounced inflammatory markers when compared to those with higher bacterial richness.[9] They also showed evidence of greater oxidative stress in the body, and, not surprisingly, a higher likelihood of leaky gut.

After the initial testing, the authors then followed their subjects for nine years and found the LGC group continued to gain more weight. But here's the good news: the researchers also found that people who increased their fiber intake from fruits and vegetables increased their bacterial richness and improved some of their health issues. That meant that people truly could welcome back more of their gut's "old friends" just by changing their diets alone.

Westernized cultures' lack of bacterial diversity is best illustrated when comparing the average gut population of Westerners to the average gut population of a people who've not yet succumbed to our modern ways. The Yanomami tribe, which lives in a remote section of mountainous tropical rain forest on the border of Venezuela and Brazil, is one of the last indigenous groups relatively untouched by civilization. They haven't been exposed to the trappings of contemporary life—they haven't eaten processed foods, taken antibiotics, or even seen a bottle of hand sanitizer. The tribespeople don't sit down to three square meals a day, but instead consume smaller meals during the daylight hours, subsisting on a diet that includes fish, wild-caught meat like venison, a variety of insects, and plenty of root vegetables covered in soil-based organisms. They also snack on bananas and drink a probiotic-rich liquid made from fermented cassava, a nutty-flavored root vegetable. Scientists found that the Yanomami's microbiome had more than 40 percent more biodiversity than the average American, perhaps the highest levels of bacterial diversity ever reported in a human group![10]

In contrast, American digestive tracts looked like barren deserts;[11] they'd lost several key foundational species. Among those missing were strains that helped metabolize carbohydrates, a strain that actively communicates with the immune system, and another known to protect humans from kidney stone formation. Stanford researchers who studied the data claimed that some of these missing microbes are at the root of many Western diseases.[12]

— We Have to Get Back to the Earth —

How did we get here? Our addiction to antibiotics is a huge driver—as is our exposure to antibacterial substances in everything from our food and water, to cosmetics, shampoo, conditioner, soap, sunscreen, makeup, and lotions, to our medicines—even our pet foods. But antibiotics are not the only danger. In our effort to sanitize our world, we have cut ourselves off from healthy bacteria in ways we are only just beginning to understand. When we put antibiotics in hand soap, we didn't make our hands much cleaner—we just made the bacteria more resistant to antibiotics.

But thanks to the dynamic field of microbiome research, we know that we can start to change our microbiome very quickly. A study of Japanese participants published in the journal *Nature* in 2010 found that the bacteria we eat and are exposed to develop a symbiotic relationship with us, the host.[13] The Japanese test group had a diet high in foods from the ocean—fish and seaweed. The researchers found that when compared with participants who lived in North America, the Japanese participants had developed specific bacteria in their digestive tracts that allowed them to better digest sushi and seaweed. The lead researcher said that consuming foods with a unique set of bacteria is like giving your body a "new set of utensils" to work with.

So does this mean we should rush to an Asian food store and start eating tons of seaweed? Not necessarily. Ideally, we should focus on consuming foods that are grown in the region where we live. The microbes found in your local soil on that piece of carrot or lettuce will help you better digest the foods in your area, while also providing your body with customized immune defense weaponry to combat pathogens you may be exposed to regularly.

Through diligent attention to increasing our diversity—in our food and supplement choices, reduced stress and medications, increased probiotics and prebiotics—we now know we can start to change our microbiome (and thereby start repairing our leaky gut) in as little as twenty-four hours. Doing so may just be the golden ticket to a world with less obesity and diabetes, fewer autoimmune conditions, less Alzheimer's and autism—even less cancer.

— Leaky Gut Hides in Plain Sight —

What makes leaky gut so difficult to diagnose is that it often hides behind some of the most debilitating conditions we face. Michelle's experience was a perfect example.

In my second year of practice, Michelle came into my clinic with her husband, John, pushing her in a wheelchair. Michelle was just thirty-five years old and had been diagnosed with fibromyalgia and chronic fatigue syndrome. In her most recent doctor's visit, her physician told her he suspected she had MS.

Michelle used a wheelchair because her chronic joint pain had become so severe that she was experiencing numbness in her extremities. She was also beginning to notice other neurological symptoms, and had grown very concerned for her future. As soon as I walked into the exam room, Michelle began sobbing. "Dr. Josh, I feel so bad," she said. "I don't think I can do it anymore."

My heart went out to her—I could see how much pain she was in just sitting there. While taking notes on her medical history and symptoms, I learned that Michelle had been a former collegiate volleyball player. She had begun to experience some stomach bloating in college, but thought it was a minor digestive issue. Then, a few years after college, she began to have abnormal bowel movements, including alternating loose stools and constipation. About five years ago, she was diagnosed with IBS—which, after two years, transitioned into total constipation. Two years before her visit, she had become exhausted and began experiencing chronic pain all over her body. Then, just in the last six months, the neurological symptoms had started. She cried quietly as she recounted her doctor's recent diagnosis of MS.

While we were talking, I also looked at the food journal that she'd brought to the office. I was immediately struck by how little fiber she ate. Her diet consisted of mostly highly refined grain products, including cereal, breads, crackers, granola, and pasta. I also noticed she had taken several rounds of prescription antibiotics while she was in college, which was about the time when her digestive problems began. I asked her about her chewing habits and, before she could answer, her husband jumped in: "Nonexistent! She pretty much swallows her food without chewing."

I suspected this detail was a big issue in her digestion. I stressed how important it was for her to chew her food thoroughly. "Ideally, we should chew thirty times per bite of food," I said. I grinned as her mouth dropped open incredulously. At the end of our consult, I wrote Michelle a prescription for tests, including a stool test, which could reveal microbial imbalance, and an organic acids test specifically looking for nutrient deficiencies.

When Michelle's tests came back, sure enough, she was severely low in several B vitamins, including folate and B_{12}, and also showed very low signs of vitamin D and zinc. The tests showed she had a major depletion in certain probiotic strains, including lactobacillus, and she had pathogenic yeast overgrowth. I knew immediately the loss of beneficial bacteria and her B vitamin deficiencies could be what was causing her MS-like neurological symptoms.

"Michelle, I have good news," I said. "I know how to help." She began following a diet high in healthy fats, vegetables, and probiotic-rich foods. I also had her begin taking a vitamin B_{12} supplement, vitamin D_3, probiotic supplements, zinc, and frankincense oil.

After just twenty-one days, Michelle was out of her wheelchair. After ninety days, she practically *strutted* into my clinic and gave me a big hug. "I can't believe it," she said. "Every one of my symptoms—all the neurological stuff, my pain and fatigue, my digestive issues—have all just disappeared." She said it felt like a miracle.

As with all of my patients, I had first looked at Michelle's digestive habits—they are usually a clear window into what's happening in the body, and they give us great information for developing treatment protocols and nutrition plans. While many people think digestive details are unimportant, in my clinic, a full digestive history is the key to solving someone's health mystery.

In fact, part of the reason you may not know much about leaky gut is simple: people generally don't love to discuss their digestive habits.

That conversation I had with my mom—in which she disclosed for the first time that she basically had been constipated for her entire life—is proof that many people don't discuss their digestive health with their doctors. We think it's embarrassing or impolite, so we keep it a secret. Over time, we come to accept and normalize gut issues that are definitely not acceptable or normal. The truth is that the gut is far from being the least civilized aspect of our anatomy; in fact, it is among the most complex, with the farthest-reaching consequences for our overall health.

Most of us have probably assumed for most of our lives that the digestive system has one simple job: to process the food we eat, extracting the nutrition and the energy we need to stay alive, and eliminating the harmful waste. But in truth, the process of digestion entails many discrete, highly intricate stages. If one of these stages gets disrupted, even a small shift could turn what should be a nourishing, fortifying process into something uncomfortable, mood altering, painful—and, in some extreme cases, harmful to the entire body.

Healing the gut (or, better yet, preventing leaky gut entirely) starts with a quick understanding of how the digestive system works best. Once we know that, we'll be better prepared to prevent it from breaking down and to restore the function of our digestive organs.

— A Trip Through Your Glorious Gut —

The star of the digestive system is the gastrointestinal tract, a hollow tube of multiple organs, stretching thirty feet long, or the height of a three-story house. Together with the GI tract, your digestion taps the liver, pancreas, gallbladder, nervous and circulatory systems, and gut microbiome. Together these organs, hormones, nerves, body fluids, and microbes combine their efforts to help us extract the nutrients from our food and drink—and end up having an enormous impact on almost every aspect of our health in the process. Let's take a brief look at this system, bit by bit, to get a frame of reference for our discussion about leaky gut.

With your first bite of food—or even your first whiff of or glance at food—saliva floods your mouth. That saliva contains the very first digestive enzyme your food encounters, which breaks down the carbohydrates as we chew. Most of us don't take that much time to chew, but chewing your food thoroughly is actually a great way to help prevent leaky gut. Chewing sends the message ahead to the stomach (to get the acid ready) and the pancreas (to send along some other enzymes to

THE WHOLE DIGESTIVE TEAM

This chart from the National Institutes of Health shows how each organ involved in digestion has its own specialty and focus.[14]

ORGAN	MOVEMENT	DIGESTIVE JUICES USED	FOOD PARTICLES BROKEN DOWN
Mouth	Chewing	Saliva	Starches
Esophagus	Swallowing	None	None
Stomach	Upper muscle in stomach relaxes to let food enter and lower muscle mixes food with digestive juice	Stomach acid	Protein
Small intestine	Peristalsis	Small intestine digestive juice	Starches, protein, and carbohydrates
Pancreas	None	Pancreatic juice	Starches, fats, and protein
Liver	None	Bile acids	Fats

the small intestines). Chewing also ensures we bite all the way *through* our food, so our digestive enzymes can access every morsel of it. By not chewing enough, not only do you miss out on nutrition still locked up in those particles, they're also more likely to make it all the way to your colon undigested—giving you indigestion and gas, and providing a generous buffet for the harmful bacterial strains that hang out there.

Once your saliva-softened food is propelled through the esophagus, it lands in the stomach. The cells in the stomach lining release hormones that keep the whole digestive system running, including producing digestive enzymes and regulating appetite. The J-shaped organ works as a mixer and grinder, its muscular walls breaking food down into a semifluid liquid known as chyme (Greek for "juice").

We tend to think of stomach acid as a bad thing, but the stomach's natural hydrochloric acid helps us. This clear, pungent solution is so powerful that it can actually be corrosive to metals, but in our bodies, it destroys harmful bacteria and helps your stomach enzymes to break down proteins. If your stomach isn't producing enough acid, you can experience acid reflux and be at a higher risk for small intestinal bacterial overgrowth (SIBO), one of the primary causes of leaky gut.

Once your stomach has mashed your chyme into the consistency of a liquid or paste, it leaves the stomach and moves into the small intestine. Well, "small" is a bit of a misnomer—when all of its twists and folds are straightened out, this amazing organ is actually twenty feet long. The pancreas, liver, and gallbladder each send some digestive juices to help the small intestine break down your food into the vitamins and minerals, proteins, carbohydrates, and fats necessary to get you through your day. If all goes well, by the time the chyme has left the small intestine and heads to the large intestine, around 90 percent of the nutrients have been extracted and absorbed.

However, sometimes things don't go as well. When you eat, the gallbladder is supposed to push bile through the bile ducts into the small intestine, where it helps dissolve fat so intestinal and pancreatic enzymes can digest them. But if you've had your gallbladder removed, your small intestine must work twice as hard to break down fats (another risk factor for leaky gut). The pancreas, a spongy, tube-shaped organ about six inches long, connects to the liver and the gallbladder via a common bile duct. When most people hear of the pancreas, they think about insulin (and maybe diabetes), but the pancreas also secretes enzymes into the small intestine that digest fats, protein, and carbohydrates. If your stomach isn't producing enough acid, or if you don't have enough digestive enzymes, food particles that haven't been properly broken down get into the small intestine. This undigested food provides *too much* sustenance for the bacteria in your gut, which can cause an imbalance in your gut microbiome, preventing proper absorption of nutrients and leading to multiple vitamin and mineral deficiencies.

When the chyme leaves the small intestine and moves into the large intestine (often referred to as the colon), most of the nutrients have ideally already been extracted and absorbed. What remains of your food (mostly fiber) stays in the colon for much longer, feeding the vast quantities of gut bacteria that live there. In fact, the microbial count climbs drastically in each stage of the digestive system, going from a few hundred in the mouth and esophagus to a thousand bacteria in our stomach, to thousands, millions, and then billions in the small intestine, until we finally get to trillions in the colon. These trillions of bacteria—including many bifidobacteria and lactobacillus genii—continue the digestive process by fermenting the fiber that remains in our food to make nutrients that feed the colon cells. This fermentation also creates short-chain fatty acids, which encourage healthy colon cell growth and support our health in many other ways. These microbes also help protect the colon from being overtaken by hordes of harmful pathogenic bacteria.

The whole process of digestion takes anywhere from twenty-four to seventy-two hours—if we're healthy. (And, as we've seen from my mom, some of our digestive processes are anything but.)

— Your Gut Barrier —

Now that you have a better understanding of how your digestive system works, let's take a closer look at the gut barrier—your intestinal lining—to understand how leaky gut develops.

The intestinal wall consumes about 40 percent of all of our body's energy. It has many functions, but the two most important are to remain open to allow the body to absorb essential fluids and nutrients into the bloodstream, and to act as a barrier that shields the body against infections and toxins. The immune system in your gut is partly responsible for this job, and so is the gut wall itself.

The gut wall has four layers: the serous layer, the muscular layer, the submucosa, and the mucosa. The outermost layer, the serous, is connective tissue, and the muscular layer is responsible for the movement that keeps food progressing through the GI tract. The mucosal and submucosal layers finish out the final layers. Together, these parts have been termed "the mucosal barrier"—the part of the gut that gets leaky.

— How a Healthy Gut Works —

When you eat, the food that enters your mouth, gets chewed up, and then travels down through the esophagus and the stomach is not really *in* your body yet—it's merely passing *through* a tunnel that stretches through the body. The place where it finally enters into your tissues and bloodstream is the mucosal barrier, this innermost layer of the gut.

The mucosal barrier controls which nutrients get absorbed while preventing allergens, microbes, or other toxins from coming in. The barrier folds over itself throughout the GI tract, increasing the surface area for digestion and absorption into the tissues—but also greatly expanding the surface area that can develop leaks. Throughout the gut, a population of beneficial bacteria and other microbes tries to keep us at that 85 percent good/15 percent bad balance. The 85 percent neutral-to-good microbiota basically act as seat-fillers on the intestinal wall to prevent harmful microbes from taking up residence. The entire time, the mucosal barrier is helping to sort out good from bad, organizing just the right level of immune response to any bad guys.

It's kind of amazing to consider how an extremely thin layer of cells can do so many important jobs at once, managing the ideal balance between the microbes that live in your gut and the immune system that protects it, shielding your entire body from incoming pathogens while also nourishing it. When things are going well, the tight junctions in the gut wall make all the right judgment calls, letting in the friends and keeping out the foes—and we don't even realize this screening process is constantly taking place. When an errant virus or pathogen does slip through the gates, our immune system snaps into action to neutralize the threat quickly. But when the tight junctions start breaking down consistently, that's when leaky gut develops.

— How We Develop Leaky Gut —

For a long time, the causes of leaky gut were largely a mystery. But in recent decades, researchers have begun to find some answers. In 2000, Alessio Fasano, MD, at the University of Maryland made a discovery that may end up changing the trajectory of autoimmunity medicine and potentially even earn him a Nobel Prize one day. Fasano isolated the only known physiological substance that directly controls the tight junctions in the gut wall, a substance he called "zonulin."[15] Making this discovery has been compared with finding the root source, sometimes called the "smoking gun," of leaky gut syndrome.[16]

Zonulin is a protein that signals the tight junctions to open and close—the only known substance in the body to do so. By controlling zonulin, scientists can open and close the tight junctions almost at will. At this point, we know of two things that can trigger the release of zonulin in the small intestine: exposure to bacteria and exposure to gluten.[17]

Infections in the gut have long been suspected as a cause of the allergic, autoimmune, and inflammatory diseases associated with leaky gut. Fasano's team discovered that when the small intestine is exposed to any infection, it secretes zonulin in response, which then basically opens the door of the tight junctions. In other words, it's possibly the zonulin, not the bacteria themselves, that directly triggers intestinal permeability.

For millennia, this zonulin response was an essential part of the body's defense mechanism—it was a way of flushing out the bad bacteria we may encounter, such as salmonella. But our modern world has drastically increased the number of triggers for zonulin, leaving the gates of our gut wide open. What was once a very healthy (and fleeting) immune system response has morphed into a never-ending cascade, causing our bodies to become chronically inflamed and vulnerable.

Many of the autoimmune conditions linked to leaky gut have a genetic component, yet researchers have determined that less than 10 percent of those with the genes for an autoimmune disease actually develop it. So why do some people with those genes get sick while others don't? The answer, put simply, is our environment. That's why the choices we make every day—the food we eat, the products we use, the stress levels in our lives, the pills we take—can make the difference between illness and health. These are all toxic microexposures that can lead to zonulin release. And these are all things, unlike genetics, that are usually within our control.

The two most significant environmental factors when it comes to the release of zonulin are:

The increase of gluten in our food supply: The hybridization of wheat, as well as its inclusion in almost all processed food products, has vastly increased our consumption of gluten, which creates conditions in the body that encourage a near-constant release of zonulin.

The increase in antibiotic usage: The rise of antibiotic medications, hand sanitizers, chemical cleaners, medications, and other microbe killers has decimated our microbial diversity. Imbalances in our microbiome have led to increases in the sheer number of bacteria crowding into our small intestine, which continues to trigger zonulin's gate-opening mechanism.

Throughout this book, we will discuss simple ways that we can reduce our leaky gut risk by addressing five core areas of our lifestyle: diet, environmental toxins born of modern convenience, stress, over-sanitation, and overmedication. The stakes are extremely high—we know leaky gut is directly linked to many serious health conditions, perhaps none as confusing and heartbreaking as autoimmune conditions. But the discovery of zonulin gives us a clear beacon of hope. Zonulin holds the key to the gut wall, and we already know the triggers for zonulin. Thus, by reducing our exposure to these triggers, and welcoming our old bacterial friends back into the gut to defend us, we can reduce our inflammation, heal our leaky gut, and possibly turn the corner of solving the autoimmune crisis in this country.

3

The Immunity Connection

A young mom walked into my clinic, holding the hand of her five-year-old son, Blake. The mother's name was Jennifer, and I could tell she was both worried and exhausted. She had been to several other physicians and was searching for a cure to the rashes that covered Blake's arms and face.

"Let me take a look," I said as I removed Blake's shirt. Poor little guy. His upper torso was just as inflamed as his arms. His skin was swollen and red.

The boy appeared to have a severe case of dermatitis, inflammation of the skin. Blake's condition was so severe that his dermatitis was threatening to blister or develop a painful crust and flake off.

"He's itchy all the time," Jennifer said. "We've seen other doctors, and they want to put him on steroids and antibiotics. That seems awfully drastic for a young boy."

A prescription-strength corticosteroid cream would be the go-to treatment of most doctors in this situation, an all-too-common example of how modern medicine treats the symptoms but overlooks the root cause of disease. After a thorough examination and discussion about Blake's health history, I concluded that the boy's body was experiencing inflammation caused by allergic reactions to the foods he ate and household toxins he was being exposed to.

I told Blake's mom that I thought he might have food sensitivities, most likely to gluten and casein, as well as allergic reactions to shampoo, the laundry detergent used to clean his clothes, maybe even the linen in his bedsheets. But to confirm my suspicions, we needed to do some testing.

I had Blake take an IgG food intolerance test and an IgE allergy test, blood and skin tests that help me zero in on the cause of immune response, and the results were not surprising: Blake was sensitive to cow's milk, gluten, strawberries, egg whites, and tree nuts and had several environmental allergies. Like so many children I'd seen, Blake's multiple food and environmental sensitivities were the outward manifestations of leaky gut.

To start addressing these issues and get the child some relief, I asked Jennifer to feed her son a gut-healing diet that included:

- ► a morning serving of fruit, such as pears or blueberries
- ► healthy fats that came from avocados, ghee (clarified butter), and coconut oil (while eliminating partially hydrogenated oils, trans fats, soybean oil, canola oil, and vegetable oil, often found in processed foods)
- ► clean protein in the form of organic grass-fed beef, free-range chicken, wild-caught fish like sockeye salmon, and collagen protein powder for his smoothies
- ► steamed vegetables, such as carrots, cauliflower, and squash

I assumed Blake's food allergies were only the tip of his inflammatory iceberg. I asked Jennifer to throw out her home-cleaning products and start over by using essential oils to clean their floors, kitchen counters, and bathrooms. I also recommended she switch out her laundry detergent, body wash, and toothpaste and replace them with homemade versions made from natural products like vinegar; baking soda; coconut oil; essential oils of peppermint, lemon, and frankincense; castile oil soap; and bentonite clay.

Three weeks later, Blake and his mom returned for a follow-up. The dermatitis that covered Blake's body and the eczema on his cheeks had disappeared. "I can't believe how quickly he got better," Jennifer said. "I'm so relieved!" We talked about how vigilance was the best defense for Blake going forward, as exposures to foods for which he'd exhibited sensitivity, or coming into contact with household chemicals like antibacterial triclosan, could kick up the same overactive immune responses. Blake's gut lining would continue to get stronger, but because his body had already generated the antibodies against those foods and chemicals, any reintroduction could trigger a relapse in his symptoms.

Blake's leaky gut had left him with a lifelong risk of excessive inflammatory response, and a predisposition to autoimmune disease. His story is a perfect example of the autoimmune crisis that is gripping our country and the world, and I hope it will give us the motivation to face our leaky gut epidemic head-on, once and for all.

— The Rising Tide of Autoimmune Conditions —

Perhaps you've recently noticed more kids like Blake, who are suffering from environmental allergies and food sensitivities. Or maybe you know several acquaintances with conditions such as celiac disease, lupus, or fibromyalgia. Maybe your dad developed Parkinson's after many years of constipation. Or your mom's memory is going downhill fast. Or your neighbor's toddler has suddenly stopped talking—and now the whole block is whispering about autism.

Maybe you recently went to the doctor to ask why you feel "off" when you eat your favorite foods these days and were shocked when the doctor said your thyroid was low and you need to start taking medication.

You are not alone. Our country is currently in the throes of an autoimmune storm. According to the *Journal of the American Medical Association*, the rate of chronic health conditions among U.S. children rose almost 15 percent between 1994 and 2006, with the largest growth among conditions believed to have an autoimmune link, such as obesity, asthma, and behavior and learning problems.[1] The *New York Times* reported that blood test analyses prove young people are five times more likely to have celiac disease today than their peers in the 1950s.[2] Type 1 diabetes among children has been skyrocketing around the world by an average of 3 to 4 percent per year—in other words, *30 to 40 percent per decade*—while the average age of onset has gotten younger. Among Finnish children today, the incidence of type 1 diabetes is five times higher than it was in the 1950s.[3] According to the CDC, food allergies among children increased *50 percent* between 1997 and 2011.[4, 5]

If considered independently, any one of these reports could be waved off as a statistical anomaly. But the simultaneous rise in the prevalence of so many medical conditions points to a larger, systemic problem. So what unites all of them?

Put simply, chronic systemic inflammation. All of these illnesses are believed to have an autoimmune basis. And they're all linked to (if not caused by) leaky gut.

Studies in respected medical journals such as the *Lancet,* the *British Medical Journal,* and the *International Journal of Gastroenterology* have suggested that leaky gut causes autoimmune diseases such as lupus and rheumatoid arthritis, and many other diverse health issues, including allergies, autism, depression, eczema, psoriasis, metabolic syndrome, and possibly many more diseases that are now being seen as autoimmune conditions for the first time. The American Autoimmune Related Diseases Association estimates fifty million Americans currently have autoimmune conditions. When compared with cancer (which affects up to nine million) and heart disease (which affects up to twenty-two million), you can see that we need a major public awareness campaign around autoimmunity and leaky gut in this country.

— What Causes Autoimmune Disease —

Autoimmune disease has long been something of a medical mystery. Researchers have struggled to understand why some people develop it and some don't, and how it can cause such dramatic, ongoing, widespread effects in the body. Now, as the pieces slowly come together, more and more clinicians and researchers are coming around to the idea that leaky gut may provide a unifying theory for most autoimmune conditions.

The theory goes like this: Before you develop leaky gut, your immune system has a very clear job. The *innate immune system* is your body's first line of defense—it acts like a watchdog, reacting quickly to any immediate threat, but not always with 100 percent accuracy. Your innate immune system helps you recover from acute injuries such as a sprained ankle and acute infections such as the common cold. The *adaptive immune system* functions more like a bloodhound or a police dog; it remembers a scent (or in this case, a pathogen) from prior exposure, and is able to identify it quickly the next time around. This immune system is activated by exposure to certain microbes. When you come into contact with a virus, your adaptive immunity "remembers" the bug, and is able to figure it out quickly at the next exposure and deal with it in an efficient manner.

This immune system is activated by immunizations. Oftentimes in today's society, when we hear the word "immunization," we immediately think "flu shot" or "vaccine"—we see them as the only way to be immunized. But natural immunizations have been around much longer—since we developed this adaptive immunity, in fact. When you're exposed to beneficial microbes from local pollen, for example, your adaptive immunity "remembers" and is able to figure it out quickly at the next exposure. That's why microexposures to pollen from local honey or walks in nature near your house help your immune system remember that particular kind of pollen, so it doesn't overreact come allergy season. In the same way, when pathogens make their way through the tight junctions in the intestinal lining, the adaptive immune system creates antibodies to neutralize them, then develops a "memory" of those bad microbes to ensure a quick response if you are ever exposed to them again.

Meanwhile, the tissue that forms part of your gut lining—your "gut-associated lymphoid tissue," or GALT—is also protecting you. Your GALT, which contains 70 percent of your immune system, faces off daily against all of the visitors that come through the GI tract, deciding who is friend or foe. All of these systems work in concert to protect you from getting sick.

But when the gut becomes permeable, all bets are off. Once zonulin, the key wielded by the antigens, opens up the gut's tight junctions, those harmful antigens make their way through the gut lining and into the bloodstream. Repeated exposure to zonulin keeps the doors wide open; soon, more and more virulent and hard-to-manage molecules start coming through, including viruses, parasites, yeast, gluten, and other troublesome food proteins such as casein—all running amok, wreaking havoc.

With the massive influx of dangerous bacteria, your adaptive and innate immune systems shift into overdrive to try to keep you safe. Your immune system stays fixed in the "on" position, blindly shooting its antibody gun at everything in its path—including your own body tissues.

Organs, such as the thyroid, get hit with friendly fire, too, creating damaged tissues and cells. Those cells need to be swept out of the body, and guess who's on the cleanup crew? The immune system, which creates specific anti-inflammatory antibodies to get rid of the mess of damaged thyroid cells. However, when this process is repeated over and over, the "cleanup" antibodies can get a little hypervigilant about cleaning up thyroid cells, and they eventually morph into "attack" antibodies—and now even healthy thyroid cells are seen as interlopers that must be eliminated. Your thyroid has become the collateral damage in the war that began at the gates of your intestines. You may only discover this when your doctor announces that you have Hashimoto's thyroiditis.

Normally the body has a system of checks and balances that keeps all of this overzealous antibody activity in line. The major player in that balance? The microbiome. A group of researchers at Caltech discovered that *Bacteroides fragilis*, a strain of "old friend" bacteria present in 70 to 80 percent of humans, helps the immune system stay in balance by supporting anti-inflammatory functions. In animal studies, the researchers proved that when *B. fragilis* is present, it basically acts as a referee, helping restore a peaceful balance between pro- and anti-inflammatory immune cells. Sadly, *B. fragilis* is one of the bacterial strains that have become endangered in recent history, which the Caltech researchers believe is directly related to our rapid uptick in autoimmune conditions.[6]

I know it sounds frightening—and it is. But there's hope. Now that we're starting to understand the source of the suffering for so many people with autoimmune conditions, we have the opportunity to stop it and vastly improve the health and longevity of our entire country at the same time. And it all starts with healing the gut.

— The Progression of Autoimmune Disease —

Now, while autoimmunity is on the rise, full-blown autoimmune conditions don't seem to happen to everyone—yet!—and that's great news. If we can figure out why some people get so sick and others don't, we can tackle autoimmunity at the source.

One of the distinguishing characteristics of both leaky gut and autoimmune disease is their progressive nature. Leaky gut typically starts off as general gut inflammation, but over time will advance to nutrient malabsorption and food or other chemical sensitivities.

Leaky Gut Progression

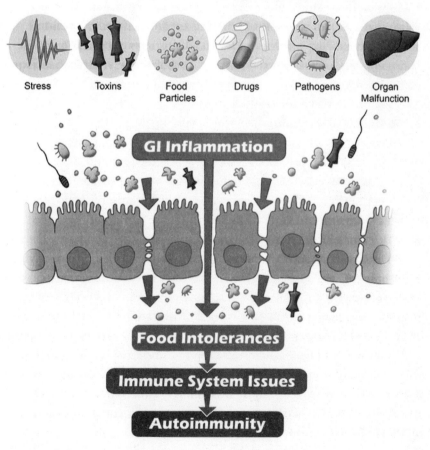

Researchers have found several common denominators that under-
lie an autoimmune disorder:[7]

1. **Genetic susceptibility:** What is your body's weak spot? Do
   neurological conditions such as MS, diabetes, or rheumatoid
   arthritis run in your family? If so, your autoimmune process
   may target your nervous system, pancreas, or joints.
2. **Exposure to inflammatory antigens:** How often have you
   been exposed to the offending microbe or entity? The list
   of these inflammatory antigens is long and growing: Does
   your diet include a lot of wheat, dairy, or other foods that
   have given you an inflammatory reaction in the past? (An inflammatory gut reaction could present itself in several ways,
   including runny nose, any digestive symptoms such as gas,
   bloating, or· upset stomach, and even low energy levels or
   fuzzy thinking.) Do you have mold in your basement? Do
   you use cleaning products and toiletries that contain harsh
   chemicals? Do you use dryer sheets, air freshener, or other
   sources of synthetic fragrances?
3. **Damaged gut lining:** Do you have a healthy and diverse microbiome, or have your beneficial bacteria been weakened
   by antibiotic use, poor diet, stress, or environmental toxins?
   Has your gut lining degraded to the point that antigens encounter no resistance from your mucosal barrier and go sail-
   ing through those tight junctions?

The sad truth is, sometimes autoimmune diseases start extremely
early in our lives. Recent research suggests antibiotic exposure during
the first few years of life can permanently reprogram the body's immune
system. An animal study at New York University found that those treated
with penicillin early in life were more likely to be overweight as adults,
with elevated fasting insulin and liver dysfunction—classic markers of
metabolic syndrome, which is now suspected to be an autoimmune
condition.[8] Another recent study from Johns Hopkins and Harvard found
that children who'd been born via C-section or who'd been treated with
antibiotics early in life had a three to three and a half times greater risk of
developing eosinophilic esophagitis (EoE), a GI condition in which white

blood cells collect in the esophagus in response to foods, allergens, or acid reflux.[9] The scariest part: EoE is a chronic immune system disease that has *only been identified within the past twenty years,* and yet the prevalence of people suffering from it has risen so rapidly that it's now considered a major cause of gastrointestinal illness.[10]

Perhaps the most unsettling aspect of autoimmune conditions is how many there are. But one thing I'd like you to take away from this discussion is that the connection with leaky gut is both a concern and an opportunity. Now that we know these connections, we can take immediate steps to feel better and to heal.

Let's consider a few of the conditions linked to autoimmunity, just to give you a sense of how widespread these conditions are. (We cannot be comprehensive here, as that would require a whole book—or several!) I sometimes find that when my patients get a sense of the scope of autoimmune conditions out there, and how leaky gut can increase their risk of developing any one of them, that information can spur them to make beneficial changes that can lead to a total transformation in their health.

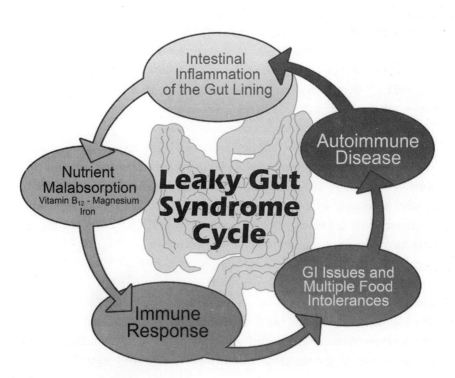

— Autoimmune Conditions and Links to Leaky Gut —

As you've no doubt heard many times when people talk about scientific research, correlation does not prove causation. We can't 100 percent definitively say that leaky gut *causes* all autoimmune disease. But we can clearly see that leaky gut makes these conditions worse. And, in many cases, the medications that help treat or relieve the symptoms of these diseases also seem to restore the gut. So whether leaky gut is the chicken or the egg, it really makes no difference—healing it may help reduce, solve, or even prevent autoimmune issues.

Celiac Disease

Celiac is the autoimmune condition with the clearest link to leaky gut. The zonulin released by gluten opens up the tight junctions of the gut lining and lets the gluten out into the bloodstream. Whereas the majority of us might need multiple exposures of gluten before the inflammatory response kicks in, for those with a genetic tendency for celiac, the immune response is triggered immediately and can have severe, even life-threatening consequences. But once gluten is removed from the diet, celiac can be resolved quickly. Zonulin decreases, the tight junctions close up, and the markers for autoimmunity antibodies start to decrease. With total abstention from all gluten, the autoimmune process shuts off, and the leaky gut—the main focus of celiac's autoimmune response—can begin to heal completely.[11]

While people with celiac disease experience an extreme immune response, even those with a gluten sensitivity are likely to struggle with leaky gut. A study at the University of Bologna found that people with nonceliac gluten intolerance had almost as much circulating zonulin as those with celiac disease.[12] Even if you don't have celiac disease, chronic exposure to gluten can harm the gut.

Diabetes

Type 1 diabetes, which once was known as juvenile diabetes, is an autoimmune disease in which the body attacks its own cells—namely, the beta cells of the pancreas—destroying their ability to make insulin.

According to the *Journal of Diabetes*, there is a strong body of evidence pointing to leaky gut syndrome as a cause of type 1 diabetes.[13]

Some research suggests that leaky gut is a preexisting condition for both type 1 and type 2 diabetes. In animal studies, leaky gut of the small intestine was present at least one month before type 1 diabetes appeared in genetically susceptible mice. Another study found that a leaky gut caused by zonulin release was detectable two to three weeks before the development of type 2 diabetes. But research suggests that if you abstain from gluten, your diabetes risk may actually plummet: animal studies that blocked the release of zonulin decreased the incidence of diabetes by 70 percent.[14]

Inflammatory Bowel Disease (IBD)

Leaky gut is a primary symptom of IBD, such as Crohn's and ulcerative colitis. Researchers have found that people typically develop leaky gut about one year before they're diagnosed with Crohn's disease— but they're still not sure if IBD triggers or is triggered by leaky gut. What they do know is, once the autoimmune process starts, it props open the door to the gut and sets up a vicious, ever-intensifying cycle of gut leakiness and inflammation.[15]

Rheumatoid Arthritis

In RA, the immune system attacks the lining of the joints throughout the body. While we're not quite sure how RA starts, we do know that the immune system plays a major role through an interaction of genes, hormones, and environmental factors. People with a specific genetic marker called the HLA shared epitope, located on a genetic site that controls immune responses, have a five times greater chance of developing rheumatoid arthritis than people without the marker.[16] Imbalances of gut bacteria, particularly infections with pathogens such as salmonella and shigella, in people with this genetic profile have been shown to trigger autoimmune reactions in the joints that damage connective tissue and cause reactive arthritis.[17, 18] People with RA also have higher levels of antibodies against certain species of intestinal bacteria, which only underscores the link between gut bacteria and RA.[19]

Psoriasis

Psoriasis is the most common autoimmune condition in the country, affecting about 2 percent of the population. When the immune system mistakenly attacks normal tissues in the body, this reaction leads to swelling and a quicker turnover of skin cells. New skin cells that usually grow deep in your skin rise to the top too quickly, piling up on top of the skin's surface, forming itchy red patches.

But the problems are not just skin deep—a third of those with psoriasis develop psoriatic arthritis, affecting the joints and the ends of fingers and toes.[20] A study of over 25,000 patients in the Kaiser Permanente Health Network, published in the *Journal of the American Academy of Dermatology*, found that people with psoriasis have twice the risk of developing other autoimmune conditions, especially those connected with leaky gut.[21] Specifically, people who have psoriasis have almost four times greater chance of developing Crohn's disease and over seven times greater chance of developing ulcerative colitis.[22] At least 36 genetic links have been found to psoriasis, including many involving innate and adaptive immunity.[23, 24]

Acne

Acne has been the bane of about 85 percent of adolescents for decades, so it's often seen as just a rite of passage for young people. The reason it is so incredibly hard to cure is its variety of causes and triggers. Some microbial colonies on the skin are involved in inflammatory acne, both making it worse and, in the case of bacteria such as staphylococcal lipoteichoic acid (LTA), making it better. LTA has been shown to reduce the amount of inflammatory cytokines released from skin cells, quieting acne's trademark swelling and redness.[25] But once the skin's microbiome has been lost or damaged, this protective mechanism is likely gone, too.

Like psoriasis, acne is not just skin deep. Researchers have begun to uncover an autoinflammatory connection with the bacteria *Propionibacterium acnes* that works the innate immune system, linking acne to classic autoimmune disease.[26] A greater number of staphylococci and a smaller number of propionibacterium (*P. acnes* in particular) were also reported in the patients with psoriasis when compared to healthy individuals.[27] Researchers believe that these similar immune pathways that are associated with the skin microbiome are linked to the development of allergies and asthma.[28]

Asthma

About 40 percent of people with asthma also have leaky gut. Food sensitivities are known triggers for wheezing in some kids with asthma, which is why researchers believe leaky gut may increase their susceptibility to allergens in their environment.[29]

Metabolic Syndrome

Long seen as a result of obesity, metabolic syndrome may soon be revealed as an autoimmune condition that *results* in obesity. In obese patients, markers for leaky gut correlate perfectly with metabolic syndrome risk factors.[30] The more zonulin in your blood, the higher your likelihood of having:

- higher BMI
- higher hip-to-waist ratio
- higher fasting insulin
- higher fasting triglycerides
- higher markers of inflammation

Considering more than one in three adults in America will develop metabolic syndrome, I think it's high time for us to get to the bottom of this one.[31]

Multiple Sclerosis

Just as the immune system's antibodies attack the thyroid in Hashimoto's disease, in multiple sclerosis (MS), antibodies attack myelin, the protective sheath around the nerves of the central nervous system. This attack causes increased permeability in the blood-brain barrier, which separates blood and other substances from flowing directly to the brain and spinal cord. When that barrier becomes permeable, proteins like gluten and toxins can pass through, causing damage to the brain and nerve tissue and resulting in neurological symptoms. According to studies, at least 25 percent of people with MS also experience increased intestinal permeability and some MS patients also exhibit the same inflammatory markers seen in patients with Crohn's disease.[32]

Autism

For a long time, even though many autistic kids had GI problems, no one was certain whether there was a cause-and-effect relationship between the two issues. Now a growing number of researchers believe that autism spectrum disorder might be better classified as an autoimmune disease, as many of the behaviors found in autism are believed to be the result of chronic inflammation that damages the blood-brain barrier, which allows particles to pass through, affecting the brain. When proteins like gluten and casein circulate in the body and reach the brain, they can cause neurological reactions in children such as poor focus, emotional outbursts, and slow cognitive development. A study published in the *Journal of Pediatric Gastroenterology and Nutrition* found that kids with autism and their relatives were more likely to have leaky gut than adults and children without autism. But once they went on a gluten-free/casein-free diet, their gut barrier function returned to normal levels, and some symptoms of autism even improved.[33]

Cancer

The immune system plays an extremely important role in helping us defend against and recover from cancer. When the body is healthy, the immune system eliminates pathogenic cells that are routinely produced by the body before these altered cells can cause any physical harm. We know that when the immune system is compromised, however, damaged cells divide quickly and often accumulate into a mass of tissue, forming a tumor.

Just one of our chromosomes, chromosome 16, holds the genes for IBD, lupus, type 1 diabetes, multiple sclerosis, and rheumatoid arthritis. All of these diseases have proven, documented links to zonulin and leaky gut. Chromosome 16 also holds the genes for autism, ALS, and polycystic ovary syndrome (PCOS)—conditions with suspected links to zonulin and leaky gut. Also on the same chromosome are genes for breast cancer, several kinds of leukemia and lymphoma, and prostate cancer.[34] As of now, there's no definitive answer about whether or not they're connected with leaky gut, but who knows where we'll be in just a few years? As researchers delve further into the connections between autoimmune conditions and leaky gut, let's hope they find some answers for cancer. In the meantime, these intriguing research connections can inspire us to take good care of the gut, so we can potentially help stop this autoimmune crisis in its tracks.

— What Autoimmune Disease Can Feel Like —

Autoimmune systems don't always announce their arrival loudly. Many people slowly develop autoimmune conditions without realizing anything is wrong. It can take about five years to get an official autoimmune diagnosis, and the average person goes to six to ten doctors before autoimmunity is recognized as the culprit, largely because the symptoms of these diseases are so disparate and vague. So it's important to be aware of the symptoms. Here are common signs of a developing autoimmune condition:

▶ Brain- and cranial-related effects include headaches, anxiety, "brain fog," and attention deficit problems.
▶ Red bumps on facial skin can be acne or rosacea. Other skin conditions such as eczema, psoriasis, and dermatitis cause red flaking skin as well.
▶ Issues in the sinus, mouth, and lungs, such as allergies, asthma, dry mouth, and frequent colds.
▶ Thyroid concerns, leading to fatigue or hyperactivity, weight gain or loss, and a general feeling of malaise or anxiety, which could be Hashimoto's disease (underactive thyroid) or Graves' disease (overactive thyroid).
▶ Joint discomfort, such as stiffness or pain, which could be a sign of rheumatoid arthritis or fibromyalgia.

- ▶ Muscle pain and weakness, or other symptoms of anemia or vitamin B_{12} deficiency, could leave you feeling drained and sore.
- ▶ Adrenal fatigue, leaving you "wired and tired," or simply exhausted.
- ▶ And finally, GI tract upset, which may indicate IBD. Stomach cramping, gas, bloating, diarrhea, and/or constipation are signs of leaky gut—and one or more autoimmune conditions could be here or just around the corner.

If you do have any of these symptoms, please don't ignore them, hoping they're nothing serious or that they'll just go away on their own.

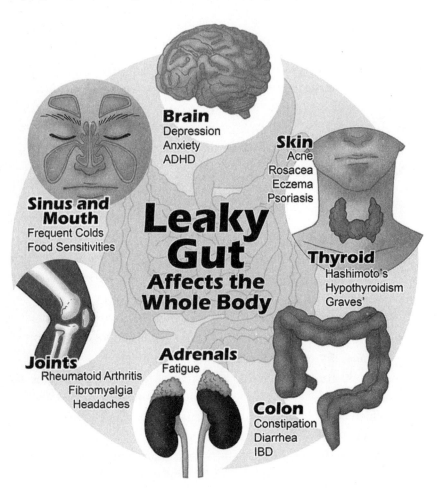

Be proactive and seek out a physician who can review your history and symptoms, preferably someone open to considering an integrative approach, such as a doctor of functional medicine. Work together to create the best autoimmune defense system for you and your gut.

While the specter of autoimmune conditions can be scary at first, we are not powerless to stop them. We *can* take control. Restoring a healthy, functioning immune system is essential to our health—and it starts with healing our gut. One of the best ways to do both—to build up our immune system and give our gut the diverse microbiome that it needs to be resilient—is through microexposures to dirt.

LAB TESTS FOR LEAKY GUT

Different autoimmune conditions require different tests for a definitive diagnosis, but a good start is determining if you have leaky gut. For definitive advanced testing, here are four lab tests to consider, all of which can be done at home:

▶ a Lactulose Breath Test (LBT), which is excellent for diagnosing small intestine bacterial overgrowth (SIBO) and leaky gut

▶ an Organic Acids Test (OAT), which reveals vitamin and mineral deficiencies

▶ an IgG (Immunoglobulin G) test, which checks for food allergies in the body

▶ a stool test, which tells you the balance of good and bad microorganisms in the body

In the resource guide at the end of the book, you will find information on how you can order these tests. While you are waiting for these results, I would not waste any time—go ahead and get started on the Eat Dirt program and specific gut type protocols in part 3. Addressing the root causes of your leaky gut now could prevent you from progressing into full-blown autoimmune disease.

4

Eat Dirt

A few years ago, my wife, Chelsea, and I were on a New York City subway on our way back to our hotel from Palma, our favorite organic Italian restaurant in Greenwich Village. We were enjoying a bit of dark chocolate when she dropped a large piece on the floor. Bummed, she bent down and picked up her piece of chocolate and put it back in the wrapper to throw away.

"It's okay. The five-second rule," I teased.

Chelsea laughed. "No way! We're on the subway."

I thought of that moment when I read an incredible study in 2015, about how the microbes found in New York City public parks, the Gowanus Canal, and subway cars were harmless—and possibly even could be healthy.

A team of DNA-swabbing researchers, led by Weill Cornell Medical College geneticist Chris Mason, identified nearly six hundred different species of bacteria and microbes on New York City subways alone, from samples taken on handrails, seat backs, floors, and closing doors. Almost half of all DNA present on the subways' surfaces matched no known organism. One subway station that was flooded during Hurricane Sandy still had the microbial profile of a marine environment.[1]

The researchers pointed to the sheer number of passengers—1.7 billion every year—as the source of the bacterial diversity. But rather than make us reach for the hand sanitizer, they said, these findings should encourage us to spend *more* time on subways, to expose ourselves to this rich microbial dirt. Mason even joked that he would advise any new parent to "roll their child on the floor of the New York subway," because exposure to germs and certain infections—especially at a young age—primes the immune system to defeat germs, viruses, and bad bacteria in the future.[2]

While I can't envision many new parents rushing to take his advice, I deeply appreciate the message behind his words. If we are ever going to slow the epidemic of leaky gut, reverse course on the autoimmune crisis, and address the rising tide of all chronic illness in the world, there's one thing we need to do more than anything else: we need to eat more dirt.

For the past century, in so many facets of our lives, we've been trying to blast bacteria. The goal was understandable: bugs bad, clean good. But in our misguided attempt to keep ourselves and our families safe, we have exposed ourselves to a growing health crisis. We have oversanitized our daily lives, and our bodies, relying on disinfectants and sanitizers, spending most of our time indoors, and rushing to get prescriptions for antibiotics any time we (or our kids) feel sick. Now we know that living in too sterile of an environment makes our bodies more vulnerable to disease, not less. In the past, scientists called this the "hygiene hypothesis"—the idea that limiting our exposure to bacteria, especially in childhood, makes us more likely to have a suppressed immune system. Now we know that what's most threatening is our modern lack of "old friends," the commensal and mutualist bacteria and other microbes in our microbiome that help fine-tune our immune responses to our environment.

By living in a squeaky-clean bubble and turning germs and dirt into villains to be destroyed or avoided at all costs, we've kept some of our most powerful allies for health at arm's length—and the devastating ramifications are piling up all around us. Researchers at the California Institute of Technology have estimated the recent *sevenfold to eightfold increase* in rates of autoimmune disorders such as Crohn's disease, type 1 diabetes, and multiple sclerosis is directly related to the lack of beneficial microbes in our gut.[3]

We've been waging our war in five main ways: oversanitizing our lives; eating processed, nonorganic foods; using modern conveniences that expose us to environmental toxins; living daily with unrelenting stress; and overmedicating. In doing so, we've ceded the battle for our microbiome and left our gut barrier wide open—and, ironically, completely vulnerable to the strains of bacteria that we were trying so hard to avoid in the first place.

I'll go over each of these five factors in detail in part 2, spelling out ways we can fight back in the five-step Eat Dirt program, as well as the five gut type protocols in part 3. But thankfully, the answer to many of our leaky gut issues is pretty simple: we just have to eat more dirt.

— Take Your Daily Dirt —

As you've read in the last three chapters, our bodies are paying the price for our modern lifestyle. Bacterial organisms have been around since the beginning of time—and the human gut has always been the first line of defense, the largest area of direct contact between us and the world.[4] Our misguided attempts to dominate nature—rather than live within it—have left us in an extremely compromised position. Thankfully, we are coming full circle. We're starting to recognize how important it is to embrace our elemental existence. Because we are literally made of mud.

If you were to take away the water in our bodies, you'd be left with mostly dirt, made of sixty of the most abundant elements in the Earth's crust.[5] This isn't such a new idea, really—it's an age-old one. The idea that humans are made from mud is foundational to many of the world's leading religions, including Christianity, Judaism, and Islam. In Christianity and Judaism, Genesis 2:7 (NLT) says, "Then the Lord God formed the man from the dust of the ground. He breathed the breath of life into the man's nostrils, and the man became a living person."

We are an amalgam of the Earth's elements: oxygen, hydrogen, carbon, nitrogen, calcium, and phosphorus, with traces of potassium, sulfur, sodium, iron, and magnesium. All of these elements come together to make a living, breathing human being. And as much as we'd like to believe we've grown much more sophisticated since the earliest days of humans, the truth is that our genome is basically the same as it was

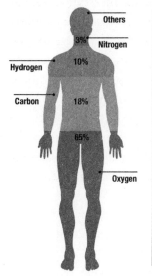

Element	Symbol	Percentage in Body
Oxygen	O	65.0
Carbon	C	18.5
Hydrogen	H	9.5
Nitrogen	N	3.2
Calcium	Ca	1.5
Phosphorus	P	1.0
Potassium	K	0.4
Sulfur	S	0.3
Sodium	Na	0.2
Chlorine	Cl	0.2
Magnesium	Mg	0.1
Trace elements include boron (B), chromium (Cr), cobalt (Co), copper (Cu), fluorine (F), Iodine (I), iron (Fe), manganese (Mn), molybdenum (Mo), selenium (Se), silicon (Si), tin (Sn), vanadium (V), and zinc (Zn).		less than 1.0

when we first appeared on Earth—while the microbiome continues to evolve *every single day.*

We have to stop seeing ourselves as the masters of the universe and eat some humble mud pie. The only way for us to coexist peacefully and healthfully with the microbes around is to simply give in and eat dirt.

Now, when I say "eat dirt," I'm not ordering you to actually scoop up a handful of soil and eat it. (Well, not exactly.) True, ensuring you get daily microexposures to soil-based organisms in dirt and other plant life *is* a part of the program. But I urge you to embrace the idea of "eating dirt" as a broader philosophy, an overarching principle I teach my patients when I talk to them about healing their gut health. It's a slightly different way of looking at the world and our place in it. And I not only preach this philosophy—I live it.

Let me tell you how I like to start the day.

Every morning around seven o'clock, rain or shine, Chelsea and I take Oakley, our Cavalier King Charles spaniel, for a twenty-minute stroll along a neighborhood path in our hometown of Nashville, Tennessee. We use this quiet time to wake up our bodies and get our blood flowing before we attack our daily schedules.

Our early walk also serves as Oakley's morning constitutional. We let him off his leash and watch him hop through mud puddles and chase after squirrels. About a half mile down the path, Chelsea and I turn around—which prompts Oakley to scamper after us.

Back home, we enter through the garage, but before I let Oakley into the laundry room and the rest of the house, I plunk myself down on the doorstep and gather him into my arms. Invariably, he's covered in something, whether it's leaves, pollen, or dirt. After fluffing his silky chestnut red-and-white coat, I grab his paws and brush off the dirt— and, with that, beneficial microbes enter the bloodstream through my skin's absorbent epidermal layer. These beneficial microbes:

- reinforce the numbers of good bacteria already in my gut
- teach those the beneficial bacteria information about responding to pathogens in the surrounding area
- aid my body in creating nutrients, including vitamin B_{12} and vitamin K_2
- support my digestion and absorption of minerals
- reduce my inflammation
- help heal (or prevent) leaky gut

I've had a dog since I was a kid, and I credit many of those walks, and much of that paw dirt, with giving me the cumulative microexposures that have helped my immune system avoid allergies. In fact, medical research has proven that having a cat or a dog as a kid cuts our risk of allergies in half.

I've become such a believer in the health benefits of getting my hands dirty that I'm constantly looking for ways to touch, feel, and yes, even *eat* dirt. My favorite way is through produce: when I purchase a fresh bunch of organically grown carrots at the farmer's market, I know I'm going to be far better off simply rinsing my carrots under running water instead of scrubbing them with a brush and some kind of produce wash, because the surface area of every carrot contains beneficial microbes. When I do this, I can take in an average five hundred milligrams of old-fashioned dirt each day, the same amount the average child consumes when playing outdoors. Five hundred milligrams, essentially the size of an average supplement capsule, may not sound like

---

THE PRICE OF CONVENIENCE

A lot of people love the convenience of bagged baby carrots—they're bite sized, prepeeled, and perfect for kids' lunches and on-the-go snacking. They also seem to stay fresh and crunchy longer than other carrots. But have you ever stopped to question why these brightly hued mini vegetables are so different from regular carrots?

Baby carrots are made by whittling down larger carrots into snack-sized chunks, which are then bathed in a chlorine solution to keep them "fresh" and shelf stable. Unfortunately, the price of this convenience is our health: the chemicals in that solution kill off beneficial bacteria in your gut.

---

much—but there are probably more beneficial microbes in that small amount of dirt than there are people living on Earth today.[6]

We *need* this dirt. Our bodies crave this dirt. And without this dirt in our diets, our health is headed in the wrong direction.

— Our Death Wish for Germs —

Our collective germophobia began 150 years ago when French chemist Louis Pasteur revealed his "germ theory" of disease, stating that germs and bugs invisible to the human eye are what make us sick. Before this, no one had ever heard of a "microbe"—no one knew that keeping clean could literally save your life. After all, living conditions in many American cities were far from sanitary a century and a half ago. Pasteur's theory revolutionized the practice of modern medicine and understanding of disease.

In the span of human history, 150 years isn't really all that much time—so when you think about it, our obsession with germs is a relatively modern phenomenon. The idea that germs around us make us sick is the reason we wash our hands after we cough, reach for our hand sanitizer after shaking hands at a business function, clean our kitchens with bleach, or throw away the stray carrot that hits the linoleum floor. It's why health-care workers practice good hygiene by washing their hands frequently and wearing disposable gloves, and surgeons use sterilized medical equipment. And while some of these measures are absolutely vital to our health—I don't think any of us wants a surgeon with dirty hands or a contaminated scalpel performing an operation on us!—our paranoia about germs has gotten out of hand. And it's not hurting the germs—it's hurting us.

Take dishwashing, for example: conventional wisdom says that we're always better off washing our glasses, plates, forks, and knives in a dishwashing machine because they get cleaner that way, because the dishes and silverware are "sterilized" by the piping-hot water. But doing so also deprives our bodies of a chance to be exposed to more bacteria, which can bolster the immune system. According to a 2015 study of over one thousand Swedish children, parents who mostly washed their dishes by hand—rather than in the dishwasher—raised children who were significantly less likely to develop eczema and somewhat less likely to develop allergic asthma and hay fever.[7] The Swedish researchers found that eating off of sanitized plates made the immune system more likely to misfire and overreact in a way that led to autoimmune conditions. In contrast, the kids who grew up without dishwashers were exposed to tiny particles of dirt and bacteria, getting repeated microdoses of immunity modulators with every meal.

Antoine Béchamp, a contemporary—and rival—of Louis Pasteur in the French Academy of Sciences in the nineteenth century, had a different take on the fundamental cause of disease. Béchamp believed disease was caused by an imbalance of good and bad bacteria in the body—if our systems were balanced, pathogenic germs could not flourish. If our ecology was imbalanced, however, bad germs could thrive. Béchamp had no way of understanding what a microbiome was back then, but he was certainly onto something. He believed that germs did not *cause* disease but were a *sign* of disease.

Well, we know which theory ended up winning the day in conventional medicine and popular culture. Pasteur's germ theory has ruled for the past 150 years. Our guiding credo ever since has been, *If you're sick, it's because you have a bug.*

How different would our world be now if Béchamp's theory had won out?

— A Spoonful of Medicine —

Until Pasteur's time, people weren't all that afraid of dirt. Think about the farmer who got hungry while tilling his fields. He'd yank an apple off the tree, brush off the skin, and chomp away.

Naturally, he was eating a little "dirt"—pollen, soil-based organisms, and other microbes—with every bite. In fact, those minute microbes actually helped to break down the polysaccharides (sugar) in the apple, making it easier to digest. That dirt on the apple also had antioxidant and preservation properties. In the era before refrigeration, it was common to store food by burying it in the ground or storing it in a dirt cellar, which helped to keep bad bacteria and yeast at bay because of the lower temperature and microbes in the soil that help preserve the food.

Most of those daily microexposures to dirt came to an end when our agrarian lifestyle tapered off during the first half of the twentieth century. People began to move from the country to the city, and while they were exposed to plenty of dirt in the city, it wasn't the beneficial, organic dirt of country living. At the turn of the century, waste management systems were in their infancy; in overcrowded cities, raw sewage flowed through the streets; people drank contaminated water; food standards were unregulated, and eating tainted or spoiled food was not uncommon; and contagious and deadly diseases spread rapidly. It makes sense that we became fearful of bugs and wanted to pasteurize our food and sanitize our homes. But today, after decades of fighting germs, the pendulum has swung too far in the opposite direction.

We've become a culture obsessed with avoiding dirt. In a nod to our germophobe forefather, we "pasteurize" some of the very products that would otherwise teem with beneficial bacteria: yogurt, apple cider vinegar, sauerkraut. Our apprehension about germs is only exacerbated when we hear about periodic *E. coli* outbreaks from tainted food (ranging from beef to tomatoes to lettuce) that generate tremendous coverage in the twenty-four-hour news cycle. It's perfectly natural and healthy to want to live in a clean home, to want to eat clean foods, and to want to be hygienic, sanitary people—but the nuclear option of germ eradication is not the way to go.

In the grand scheme of things, we need *more* microorganisms, not fewer. The specter of those *E. coli* attacks may hang over us while we spray antibacterial solutions on our kitchen countertops, but that mis-placed fear has left our systems more vulnerable than ever. Introducing more beneficial microbes into our lives, at every step, can improve the balance of bacteria in the gut, preventing dangerous strains from mak-ing their way in and giving the good microbes the numbers they need to defend the gut lining. Remember—those good microbes are not only our best defense against the zonulin-triggering bad bacteria that loosen up the tight junctions in the gut barrier, they also teach our immune system to stand down when those molecules do get through, helping us avoid autoimmune conditions. If we can refortify those missing good old bacterial friends, we can reboot our own personal microbiome, and begin to heal the gut.

— An Idea as Old as Dirt —

The idea of eating dirt has also been around a long time, dating from Hippocrates more than twenty-five hundred years ago. You name the civilized culture in past millennia, and you'll find a record of those people consciously including a bit of dirt in their diets.

In cultures around the world, pregnant women often crave dirt or clay—and some actually eat it. In sub-Saharan Africa, pregnant women eat dirt during the first, second, or third trimesters, often several times a day. The dirt has a soothing effect on the stomachs of those fighting morning sickness as well as providing vitamins and minerals that their changing bodies crave. Certain types of soil, especially clay, are high in iron and sulfur, which pregnant women naturally long for because their bodies are demanding more hemoglobin—the protein in red blood cells that carries oxygen to the cells—to produce blood for a developing baby.[8]

But perhaps most interesting is what the dirt does for the baby's im-mune system: researchers found that eating dirt creates IgA antibodies in the mother that immunize the fetus against common antigens during pregnancy. Those same IgA antibodies flow in her breast milk and help line the gut of the newborn baby. Traditional cultures may not have known exactly *why* dirt was good for them, but clearly, that dirt did a body good.

More specifically, pregnant women sometimes crave clay, which—

as any fourth-grader could tell you—is different from regular dirt because of its denser nature and tiny soil particles. Clay has unique microbes that are excellent for the gut but also bind toxins and help pull them out of the body. One of the most popular and healthiest clays to eat is bentonite clay, which is composed of volcanic ash. When I have patients struggling with loose stools or diarrhea, I always suggest they take a teaspoonful of bentonite clay in a glass of water twice every day until they experience relief.

I'll never forget our Caribbean honeymoon in St. Lucia several years ago for a variety of reasons, but one memory that stands out is when Chelsea and I signed up to take a mud bath together at a nearby volcano where hot, muddy water flowed out of the side of a mountain. We were told by the locals to submerge ourselves in the mud and then let it dry and stay on our skin for thirty minutes before washing off. We followed their advice and covered ourselves from head to toe, then relaxed and gave the mud time to dry. Afterward, we not only felt rejuvenated but our skin was positively glowing from the generous dose of healthy microbes in Caribbean mud.

Like human cells, microbes die or "slough off," which means they need to be replenished on a regular basis. When we're intentional about getting our hands dirty and eating dirt every day, we give our bodies progressive immunity boosters and a better chance of maintaining that 85-to-15 percent balance of beneficial bacteria and pathogenic bacteria. That's a lot of good bacteria that we need to seek out on a daily basis.[9] It didn't surprise me when our guide told us that any time locals come down with an illness, they take a soak in the mud to get their health back on track.

— Missing Out on Vitamin Dirt —

We used to have backyards filled with vegetable gardens and flower beds that put us in close contact with good earth when we planted and hoed and weeded.

These days many people live in subdivisions where every house has a backyard the size of a racquetball court, landscaped with paving stones and devoid of any greenery. Others live in high-rises, condominium complexes, or apartment blocks in urban areas, without a plot of dirt or blade of grass in sight.

Kids also aren't getting dirty like they used to. Part of that comes from our collective obsession with sanitizing hand gels, antibiotic soaps, and germ-killing wipes. But very few kids are allowed to roam neighborhoods or play in the woods anymore. Instead of playing hide-and-seek in the bushes or digging foxholes for "army" games, playtime for most elementary school–age kids now consists of sitting inside and staring at a variety of screens.

Contrast that with our grandparents' generation, when many children and teens had to complete chores around the farm before and after school: gathering eggs, shoveling the compost pile, weeding the garden, feeding animals. Our parents' generation got their hands dirty as kids, too—who hasn't heard stories about their dad or uncle mowing lawns or raking leaves to make some pocket money? But as technology has improved our lives and outsourcing household chores has become easier and cheaper, we've lost contact with these basic routines. I remain nostalgic for a simpler time—a more humane pace, living in tune with the rhythms of the sun and the seasons, breathing in the smells (and microbes) of organic soil every day, being connected with our neighbors, animals, families, and the land. That way of life worked well with so many aspects of our core biological and social needs—and, not coincidentally, also encouraged our microbiome to thrive.

We can't reverse time, of course, and we are lucky to be living in an era of such incredible progress. But all of that progress comes with a price, and we must be mindful not to get rid of the benefits along with the problems. We can add facets of that earlier, simpler lifestyle back into our days, and in doing so we will benefit not only physically, but also emotionally and spiritually, and help heal our ailing guts in the process.

— It's More Than Just Dirt —

Good bacteria abound in almost every setting and substance in nature. Throughout the rest of this book, we will look at hundreds of ways you can add "dirt" to your life, boosting your immune system and populating your gut with good bacteria. In the Eat Dirt program in parts 2 and 3, I'll also guide you in selecting which dirty practices would work best with your own constitution and lifestyle.

Once you start looking, you'll find countless ways to bring vital practices into your life. For example, on any given day, you could:

▶ **Eat probiotic-rich foods like kefir, yogurt, and sauerkraut:** One of the reasons many people today are lactose intolerant (or have an allergy to dairy products) is that pasteurization kills off the beneficial probiotics and enzymes. According to several published medical studies, when someone with lactose intolerance consumes a dairy product that is raw or fermented—which is also higher in probiotics or enzymes—symptoms of lactose intolerance can diminish. Kefir is especially beneficial, and a study in the *Journal of the American Dietetic Association* showed that kefir improves lactose digestion and tolerance in adults with lactose malabsorption.[10]

▶ **Consume raw honey and bee pollen:** Many of us develop seasonal allergies because we don't spend much time outside and only have periodic exposure to pollen. But bee pollen, which worker bees collect on their bodies as they go to and from the hive, is also effective against a wide range of respiratory diseases. In a study published in the *Journal of Pharmaceutical Biology*, researchers found that a mixture of raw honey and bee pollen showed a significant reduction in inflammation, improvement in immune function, and protection for the liver.[11] An independent case study conducted at a medical clinic in Denver reported that 94 percent of patients were completely free from allergy symptoms once treated with an oral regimen of pollen. These gradual and natural immunizations from the microbes in the honey and pollen take up residence in your gut and help modulate your immune system to adjust to the local environment. Honey also provides an excellent source of prebiotics, to nourish the gut bugs as it educates them. Eat local honey throughout the year, and when allergy season arrives, you'll already have had a healthy exposure and your immune system will be less likely to overreact to the extra pollen in the air.

▶ **Get a dog.** A study appearing in the medical journal *Clinical and Experimental Allergy* showed that having pets may improve the immune system and reduce allergies in children. The researchers studied 566 children with pets, including dogs and cats, taking blood samples when the children turned eighteen. They found that children who had cats had a 48 percent decrease in allergies, and those with dogs had a 50 percent decrease in allergies.[12] The explanation? An animal that plays in the dirt brings diverse microbes into the home, some of which the kids may breathe in and others that enter through the skin from touching their furry friends. These microexposures may be in very small doses, but they add up over time and help populate the good microbes in your gut, boosting immunity—which is exactly why I don't mind cleaning Oakley's dirty feet.

▶ **Swim in the ocean:** You've probably heard or experienced for yourself how a cut seems to heal quickly after a dip in the ocean. Part of that is due to the salt content of the water, but the good microbes and bacteriophages present in salt water also have therapeutic merit. A 2013 study in *Seminars in Arthritis and Rheumatism* found that those who took baths in minerals salts from the Dead Sea had a decrease in skin inflammation, rheumatoid arthritis, and psoriasis.[13]

▶ **Get grounded:** Just the simple act of putting your bare feet on the ground can affect your health in several surprising ways. When you stroll barefoot on grass, dirt paths, shoreline sand, or even concrete sidewalks after a rainstorm, the soles of your bare feet come into direct contact with the surface of the Earth, creating the opportunity for billions of bacteria and other beneficial microbes to catch a ride. Researchers have become so fascinated with the health benefits of walking barefoot that it's given rise to a whole new field of study on the practice, now being called "earthing" or "grounding." A study in the *Journal of Environmental and Public Health* found that the Earth's negative charges can literally "ground" us, similar to a grounding wire of an electrical tower. The connection between our skin and the Earth's surface may help to stabilize our internal bioelectrical environment in a way that regulates the normal functioning of our body systems. Researchers believe this exchange of electrical charge may factor into setting the biological clock, regulating circadian rhythms, and balancing cortisol levels. A 2006 study published in the *Journal of European Biology and Bioelectromagnetics* found that after participants engaged in earthing, their cortisol levels reverted to normal levels and rhythms, rising in the morning and falling in the late afternoon.

Several other studies on earthing have been conducted and found promising results for a better night's sleep, higher energy levels, decreased inflammation, and reduced pain. Just kicking off your shoes and walking on the ground for a few minutes every day could help you absorb this beneficial combination of electrical currents and microbes (or what I like to call "vitamin G").

▶ **And, yes, literally eat dirt:** As we've discussed, soil-based organisms (SBOs) support gut health and immune response. Why, exactly? In the plant world, SBOs help plants grow. Without their protection, otherwise healthy plants become malnourished and are susceptible to disease or contamination by fungi, yeasts, molds, and candida. Just as plants grow best in healthy soil teeming with highly active microorganisms, you, too, need these organisms to live a long, healthy life.

More than eight hundred studies exist in the scientific literature that reference soil-based organisms. Their common denominator is that they link SBOs to successfully treating a wide variety of health conditions, including:

- ▶ allergies
- ▶ asthma
- ▶ irritable bowel syndrome
- ▶ ulcerative colitis
- ▶ flatulence
- ▶ nausea
- ▶ indigestion
- ▶ malabsorption
- ▶ nutrient deficiency
- ▶ autoimmune disease

▶ inflammatory disease

▶ bacterial, fungal, and viral infections

See any connections there?

Throughout the first four chapters, we've looked at how these conditions are all linked to leaky gut. We now know that SBOs nourish cells in the colon and liver and actually create new compounds such as B vitamins, vitamin K$_2$, antioxidants, and enzymes. SBOs can destroy or crowd out harmful pathogens such as candida, fungi, and parasites. They also kill off bad bacteria that can bind to or puncture the gut wall. And like clay, they have been shown to bind to toxins and extract them from the body. SBOs also help to regulate the immune system and naturally reduce inflammation in the gut and throughout the entire body.

Perhaps one of the best dirt-based supplements is shilajit— pronounced *shee-lay-jit*—which comes from dense, nutrient- and mineral-rich soil high in the Himalayan mountains bordering India and Tibet. Shilajit contains at least eighty-five minerals, including two of my favorites—humic acid and fulvic acid—that are commonly used as a soil supplement in agriculture. Fulvic acid and humic acid help the body transport minerals through thick cell walls and prolong cell life.

Over the years, I've seen hundreds, if not thousands, of patients get remarkable results by supplementing their diets with soil-based organisms. One of them was a woman named Carolyn.

A fifty-eight-year-old grandmother, Carolyn was fifty pounds overweight. Around the time of her first visit, her self-esteem was at an all-time low. She also suffered from memory problems, insomnia, depression, and fatigue.

Throughout our conversation, it was clear to me that her adrenal and thyroid glands were desperately in need of support, which I advised she get from a diet centered on organic vegetables and fruit as well as fermented foods. I advised her to stop eating gluten and processed sugar, which wasn't going to be easy for her, as she ate a lot of processed carbohydrates. But Carolyn was so determined to regain her health that she willingly gave them up. My other major recommendation was to take a nutritional supplement with an SBO probiotic.

In the first thirty days of following this protocol, Carolyn lost eighteen pounds. With her digestive system receiving all of this supportive reinforcement, her body had the resources it needed to reshape itself and regain a healthier form.

Very soon, Carolyn had lost seven inches off her waist and nine inches off her hips. She had more energy than ever before, and was finally motivated to exercise. She told me she was enjoying life more fully than she had in years.

The changes experienced by Carolyn are almost identical to those I've seen in many other patients who follow a similar regimen. Once they focus their attention on eating dirt—literally and metaphorically, in what they eat and how they live—health issues that have plagued them for years often disappear, sometimes in less than thirty days.

In America, we've come to expect that it will take a lot longer to solve these health issues, but that only goes to show you that when you're intentional about increasing beneficial microbes in your gut, your gut takes care of you. And taking nutritional supplements with soil-based organisms could be one of the most important aspects of "eating dirt."

— Time to Get Back to the Land —

The author William Bryant Logan once wrote in a piece for the *New York Times* that dirt is the "ecstatic skin of the earth," a life-sustaining substance that should be treated with care and respect. I couldn't agree more.

We've spent the past century acting like we have the upper hand in nature. It's time to recognize that this isn't a fight we want to win. We humans are vastly outnumbered by our microbial friends. We need to call a truce, to lay down our weapons, and to recognize that resistance is futile—we can't defeat our bugs, and we shouldn't want to. The more we strive to live harmoniously on the Earth, in the dirt, and with our microbiome as good fellow citizens, the more our good old friends, those trillions of beneficial bacteria, will be all too happy to help heal our guts and make us whole again.

What do you say—are you ready? *It's time for us to eat dirt!*

— part two —

THE FIVE
FACTORS OF
GUT HEALTH

5

You Are What You Eat

I f we were able to consistently choose better-quality foods—to ditch the processed stuff with all of its chemicals and sweeteners and simply eat a little bit closer to the source (as in, the dirt)—most of our gut issues would be resolved. In this chapter, we'll discuss the first of the worst gut grenades: the modern American diet. Let's take a look at some of the most gut-devastating ways in which our diet has been dragged away from its dirty origins, and how we might get back to eating close to the soil once more.

— Supersizing the Bad Guys —

Around the same time that I was studying to become a doctor of functional medicine, the documentary *Super Size Me* was released. In it, filmmaker Morgan Spurlock chronicled his journey of eating three meals a day at McDonald's every day for one month. At the end of this experiment, his weight had ballooned by thirty pounds, his blood pressure had skyrocketed through the roof, his cholesterol levels had shot up sixty-five points, his liver had gone into toxic shock, his energy level had dipped to a listless state, his skin had the pallor of gray meat, and his girlfriend complained about their sex life.

Super Size Me initiated a national conversation on junk foods and their toxic mix of carbohydrates, bad fats, chemicals, and preservatives. The documentary jolted mainstream audiences awake from their processed food comas and became a turning point for the fast food industry, which stopped its ubiquitous practice of supersizing and began to offer more salads.

I always wondered what was going on inside Spurlock's microbiome when he went on his thirty-day McDonald's binge. How did his gut react to such an onslaught of toxic food? Thanks to Tim Spector, a professor of genetic epidemiology at King's College in London, we now have some idea.

Spector was intrigued by a study published in the medical journal *Diabetes* in which lab mice given an intense high-fat, high-sugar diet experienced weight gain, diabetes, inflammation, and increased intestinal permeability (or, as we know it, leaky gut).[1] The mice's microbiota, devastated by the horrible diet, had undergone a lasting change to their ecosystem. Spector wondered how the human body would react under the same circumstances, but making a group of people sick on purpose is hardly ethical. Instead, he tracked down a University of Pittsburgh study that was illuminating.[2]

The study had observed the diets of two different groups of people: twenty African Americans and twenty rural black South Africans. Before the study, the African American participants had been eating a typical American diet—a lot of fried foods and very few fruits and vegetables—while the South Africans had always consumed a traditional local diet high in beans and vegetables. For two weeks, the groups swapped diets, with the South Africans eating burgers, fried chicken, and fried potatoes. Spector found that after a diet high in fat and animal protein but low in dietary fiber, the South Africans experienced remarkable changes in their biomarkers that indicated colon cancer risk. The blood work showed that their health had taken a serious decline—in just two weeks!

The African American group, however, experienced positive changes. After two weeks of consuming corn porridge served with vegetables, beans, or a meat stew, their biomarkers for colon cancer were greatly reduced.

Wanting to investigate further, Spector made a deal with his son,

Tom: he would buy him McDonald's meals every day for ten days, if he could study Tom's microbiome afterward.

For ten days at every meal, Tom ate a Big Mac or Chicken McNuggets, plus the obligatory fries, all washed down with a Coke. He collected stool samples before, during, and after his fast food regimen. He became weak, and friends told him he'd developed a strange gray color. "I really felt unwell," he said. "When I finally finished, I rushed to the shops to get some salad and fruit."[3]

Teams from Cornell University and the British Gut Project tested Tom's microbiome, and the results were startling: his community of gut microbes had been devastated. Tom lost fourteen hundred species of microorganisms—nearly 40 percent of his total!—in just ten days. His gut didn't recover right away, either; it was months before beneficial microbes repopulated his gut.

But it's not just the obvious junk food offenders that can have such a serious impact on your gut health. Many of the packaged foods on supermarket shelves labeled as "healthy" lay waste to our microbes, with various ingredients and additives directly contributing to leaky gut. A recent article in *Autoimmunity Reviews* drew a direct line between industrial food additives, leaky gut, and autoimmunity, citing added sugar and salt, emulsifiers such as polysorbate 80 or lecithin (commonly found in ice cream, chewing gum, and even some vitamins), and gluten as big offenders.[4]

Canola oil and other vegetable oils widely used in salad dressings and cooking oils are also major culprits of gut dysfunction, as they have been shown to eviscerate many of our beneficial microbes. A study published in the *American Journal of Clinical Nutrition* found that consuming hydrogenated oils greatly increases inflammation throughout the entire body.[5] Deli meats are another common offender. They're loaded with gluten, hydrogenated fats, and nitrites, which can lead to digestive troubles for many people. A 2008 study in *Nutrition and Cancer* demonstrated that people who consume processed meats have a greater risk of cancer,[6] and in 2015, the World Health Organization's International Agency for Research on Cancer (IARC) categorized processed meat as equivalent to cigarettes and asbestos in terms of cancer risk. Not even microwave popcorn is as safe as you might assume: a statement released by the U.S. Food and Drug Administration announced that microwave popcorn contains perfluorooctanoic acid (PFOA), a synthetic chemical found in nonstick pans that's been linked to cancer and hormone disruption.[7]

Very few people are aware of how the foods they eat affect their gut, or create a constant tug-of-war between harmful bacteria and good bacteria inside their digestive tracts. We need to become more mindful that the foods of the modern world—even many of the ones we've long considered to be "healthy"—are making us sick.

— Old Favorites, New Foes —

Sometimes old eating habits die hard, even for people who should know better. In the lead-up to the 2012 Olympic Games in London, I was charged with helping our nation's best swimmers reach peak performance in a sport where the difference between gold and silver can be the length of a fingernail. Ask Michael Phelps, who won his seventh gold medal at the Beijing Games in 2008 by one-hundredth of a second in the hundred-meter butterfly.

One of the swimmers I worked with was Cullen Jones, a fifty-meter and hundred-meter freestyle sprinter who was coming back from a shoulder injury he suffered during a weight-lifting exercise. We were chatting poolside one day when I asked him what his training diet was like.

Cullen reflected a moment. "Well," he said, "the staff nutritionist has me drinking Nesquik chocolate milk after every workout."

Chocolate milk? I would later learn this is quite common, but I pretended not to be shocked as I urged him to continue telling me about his diet. He said that he usually ate peanut butter and jelly sandwiches and drank chocolate milk—a favorite among many of the athletes—all day long at the training facility. When he was on his own, he grabbed a meal at McDonald's or Burger King.

Okay, one step at a time, I thought. The first thing I needed to do was wean Cullen off chocolate milk, a mixture of homogenized, pasteurized milk with heaping teaspoons of white sugar and refined cocoa. Since Cullen wasn't progressing like everyone had hoped, the team nutritionist gave me permission to try something new. I met again with

Cullen and said I'd like him to start consuming a superfood smoothie for breakfast using coconut milk, blueberries, and an organic protein powder. He readily agreed to make the switch.

That one change—from chocolate milk to healthy smoothies—helped me rehab Cullen's shoulder much faster using the physical therapy exercises, chiropractic adjustments, and deep tissue massages I gave him.

After seeing great results with Cullen, the coaches requested that I begin working with other U.S. Swim Team members, such as Michael Phelps, Ryan Lochte, Peter Vanderkaay, and Missy Franklin. I was more than happy to comply.

Competitive swimming is a highly demanding physical endeavor, and Michael was famous for saying that he burned through twelve thousand calories a day—but let's just say that they weren't the healthiest twelve thousand calories in the world. Ryan admitted that he was a junk-food fanatic who'd eat a whole bag of potato chips before diving into the pool and head straight to McDonald's after his early morning workout for three Egg McMuffins, hash browns, and a chicken sandwich!

I suggested to Ryan that he swap out his junk food breakfast for scrambled organic eggs, oatmeal, and fresh fruit. For lunch and dinner meal options, I suggested he eat salads and healthy wraps that contained clean sources of protein. After Ryan won two golds, two silvers, and one bronze medal in London, I remember him telling the media that his diet had improved greatly since the 2008 Summer Games. "Our diet became a bigger focus for us," he said, speaking about the U.S. Swim Team. "I'm not sure it made a big difference in our swimming, but it sure made a big difference in our recovery."

The foods we eat affect our well-being, not just on a cellular level, but on a whole-life level—how we feel, how much energy we have, how strong we are, how capable we can be. So let's take a look at the top offenders when it it comes to the foods that hurt the gut and set us up for disease. While a complete list would be much longer, I want to focus here on the foods that seem to be the favorites of many of my patients, and offer you safe alternatives. I urge you to read through this list and identify the foods that might be causing you digestive harm, and then abstain from eating those foods, even for just a few weeks. I've seen firsthand the impact these "gut grenades" have on the digestive tract—and it's not pretty.

— The Dairy Dilemma: Cow's Milk —

As a kid, I loved drinking milk. It was a part of all of our childhoods, wasn't it? When I was going through a growth spurt, I must have drunk a half a gallon a day. But while studying to become a physician, I learned some things about milk that gave me pause. The more I learned, the more I was convinced that milk was not the answer to healthy bones and muscles—but what was?

Altering the *type* of dairy I was consuming.

The health of the animal and the processing methods of milk can categorize dairy as either one of the healthier foods in the world or one of the worst. If you're consuming milk, yogurt, butter, and cheese produced from conventionally raised cows that are fed a steady stream of antibiotics, your dairy intake may be playing a role in antibiotic resistance. Not just for you, either—also for your family and everyone else in the community. Conventional dairy may also increase your risk of being overweight and even of getting cancer.

The pasteurization process that most conventional dairy products undergo destroys essential enzymes and probiotics, as well as alters vital amino acids. Nearly all commercial milk is also homogenized, a process that oxidizes fats and creates free radicals. Free radicals are unstable oxygen molecules that are known to weaken the immune system and result in intestinal inflammation, leading to leaky gut.

According to a study published in the *Journal of Agricultural and Food Chemistry*, a single glass of pasteurized milk can contain up to twenty different chemicals. We know that growth hormones and antibiotics are regularly fed to cows, but researchers at the University of Jaen in Spain also found traces of numerous drugs such as niflumic acid, mefenamic acid, flunixin, diclofenac, ketoprofen, and ibuprofen, which are commonly used as painkillers for the animals.[8] Everything these cows get injected with goes straight into their milk. This is important because the oxidized fats present in homogenized milk often pass through the gut wall, carrying the hormones, steroids, drugs, and other compounds into the bloodstream and off to the rest of the body.

I rarely consume cow's milk because even organic versions in this country tend to contain a protein called A1 beta-casein. The result of a relatively recent genetic mutation, this protein is more common among the Holstein cows of American and some European industrial dairies, and can be more inflammatory to the body than gluten. A1 beta-casein releases beta-casomorphin-7, an opioid with a structure similar to that of morphine that's been linked to autism and schizophrenia. This protein may also create a shortage of antioxidants in the brain, which is another risk factor for autism.[9]

Cows whose milk contains only A2 beta-casein protein, the older version of the protein, are typically bred in the Middle East, Africa, India, and New Zealand and can be difficult to find in America and Europe. Because of this, I recommend choosing **raw cow's milk dairy products from only Jersey or Guernsey cows**, when you can find them.

In contrast to cow's milk, the dairy I personally drink and recommend to all my patients is **raw, organic, fermented, and typically made from goat and sheep milk**. Few foods in the world contain the nutritional array of probiotics, omega-3 fatty acids, protein, calcium, magnesium, and vitamin K_2 that these raw dairy products do.

Most Americans grow up consuming only cow's milk, which has a mild taste, while goat's milk has a strong, distinctive taste. Even if you think you don't like goat's milk, I urge you to give it another try. Especially goat's milk kefir, which is incredibly healthy for the gut and offers numerous benefits for the body. Goat's milk is lower in lactose, or milk sugars, than cow's milk; when fermented, it may not contain any lactose at all. The fatty acids in goat's milk are easily burned for energy, so they are not stored as fat. These fatty acids help lower cholesterol levels and have been shown to be beneficial for conditions such as cardiovascular disease and intestinal disorders.

Sheep's milk is creamier and less tangy than goat's milk with a higher fat content. Unfortunately, sheep's milk can be harder to find. But sheep's milk cheese—such as feta from Greece, Roquefort from France, and Manchego from Spain—is delicious.

If, for whatever reason, you can't bring yourself to consume fermented goat's milk or sheep's milk, you can also make a switch to one of two plant-based alternatives, coconut or almond milk:

Coconut milk, with its creamy texture and slight natural sweetness, should be much more popular than it is. This gut-friendly beverage actually isn't "milk" at all—it is a combination of the white liquid inside a fresh coconut blended with coconut meat and then strained, resulting in a thicker coconut "milk."

Coconut milk has an amazing nutritional profile and is a miracle beverage when it comes to gut health. It contains lauric acid, a beneficial medium-chain fatty acid, and is believed to have antibacterial, antifungal, and antiviral properties, which all help prevent leaky gut. Even though coconut milk's fatty acids are primarily saturated fats, they lower cholesterol levels, improve blood pressure, and prevent heart attacks and stroke. And because coconut milk is completely free from dairy, lactose, soy, nuts, or grains, it's a great option for anyone with food allergies.

Almond milk is another dairy-free milk substitute that is becoming more popular as more and more people discover its creamy texture and nutty taste. A serving of almond milk contains 50 percent of the recommended daily amount of vitamin E, an antioxidant essential for skin health. Almond milk also contains monounsaturated fats and is high in omega-3 fatty acids, which can help to lower levels of bad LDL cholesterol and support cardiovascular health. Additionally, almond milk is high in the amino acid L-arginine, which is great for anyone looking to get fit or put on healthy lean muscle. Almond milk can be a godsend to those with gut issues triggered by lactose intolerance.

— Grain in the Gut —

Wheat is the most commonly used grain and the predominant ingredient in everything from breakfast cereal to bagels to pasta, pizza, and desserts. While it's true that people have been baking and cooking with wheat for centuries, today's wheat does not resemble the wheat of our ancestors. For the last fifty years, modern wheat has been hybridized, crossbred with other grains and species to increase yields,

L-GLUTAMINE HEALS LEAKY GUT

L-glutamine is one of the best supplements for leaky gut. Synthesized by the body from glutamic acid or glutamate, L-glutamine is a fuel source for the cells in the small intestine. L-glutamine also helps moderate the body's IgA immune response, an antibody associated with food sensitivities and allergies. A study of twenty postoperative patients in the *Lancet* found that supplementing with L-glutamine helped maintain the health and length of intestinal villi as well as preserve the mucosal lining and prevent further worsening of leaky gut.[10]

If the body is unable to produce enough, it needs to get it directly from your diet. While L-glutamine can be found in animal proteins such as meats and dairy, beans, raw spinach, parsley, and red cabbage, it is known as a conditionally essential amino acid, because it is used by the body in large amounts. That's why L-glutamine supplements are so critical for people with leaky gut. If you are looking to improve digestive health and heal leaky gut I recommend you take 5 grams of glutamine powder twice daily with meals.

and sprayed with massive amounts of chemical fertilizers and pesticides. (The USDA Pesticide Data Program found traces of sixteen pesticides on wheat flour during a 2004 study.)[11] There's been another cost to this hybridization process: fewer nutrients, more weight-producing carbohydrates, and more gluten, phytic acid, and amylopectin. In my opinion, our wheat consumption is the primary culprit of our country's obesity epidemic.

Gluten, a protein found in wheat, rye, spelt, and barley, is derived from the Latin word for "glue," which makes sense because this sticky, gooey protein acts like an adhesive to hold foods together. Gluten in a flour-and-water mixture gives dough its elastic qualities and allows bread to rise during the baking process. Yet we lack the specific enzymes to fully break down and absorb gluten. Large blocks of undigested protein find their way into the small intestine, where they slow the absorption of other valuable nutrients. Our immune systems view gluten as foreign bacteria and react en masse, causing collateral damage to the intestinal wall in the process, creating the perfect conditions for zonulin to unlock the wall's tight junctions. As you learned earlier, those gluten molecules sail right through the intestine, priming us for a variety of diseases and digestive troubles.

Phytic acid is considered an "antinutrient"—a naturally occurring substance found in plant foods that blocks the absorption or proper functioning of other nutrients in the body. This mineral binder prevents our bodies from absorbing key bone-building nutrients such as calcium, magnesium, iron, copper, and zinc, which creates nutrient deficiencies and reduces the digestibility of starches, proteins, and fats. It can be found on the bran of all grains as well as the outer coating of seeds and nuts, and is an enzyme inhibitor. When grains are unsprouted and unfermented, the phytic acid can irritate the intestines and cause leaky gut.

Grains also contain amylopectin, which has been called a "super carbohydrate" for its ability to increase blood sugar faster than other carbohydrates. (In this case, "super" is not a good thing.) The molecular structure of amylopectin causes this starch to be more easily digested than other complex sugars, which raises blood sugar levels faster than you can say, "Sure, I'll have a sandwich."

In a study from the *American Journal of Clinical Nutrition*, participants were given a diet that was 70 percent amylopectin or 70 percent amylose, a different but healthier "resistant" starch that isn't as quickly digested as amylopectin. Because it takes longer to break down, amylose is fermented by bacteria in the large intestine similar to how some types of fiber are broken down—a process that limits spikes in blood sugar levels, lowers cholesterol, and feeds the beneficial bacteria in the colon.[12] Foods rich in amylose tend to have a low glycemic index: fruits, vegetables, salads, and organic whole-grain products. In contrast, foods with amylopectin have a high glycemic index: white breads, starchy potatoes, and sugary desserts. The study found that those on the amylopectin diet had high glucose and insulin responses after a meal, which led to fat storage on the body, specifically in the abdominal area, otherwise known as belly fat. Stick with the amylose!

A lot of people have a hard time giving up breads and baked goods, but the good news is, you don't have to abstain from these treats forever just because you're eliminating gluten from your diet. The

---

DIGESTIVE ENZYMES HELP SOOTHE TROUBLED GUTS

The phrase "you are what you eat" is a fallacy. As I always tell my patients, "you are what you digest." And digestive enzymes are key to both better digestion and nutrient absorption.

If you have any type of digestive disease, such as acid reflux, gas, bloating, leaky gut, irritable bowel syndrome (IBS), Crohn's disease, ulcerative colitis, diverticulitis, malabsorption, diarrhea, or constipation, then digestive enzymes can help. Digestive enzymes can take stress off the stomach, pancreas, liver, gallbladder, and small intestine by helping break down difficult-to-digest proteins, starches, and fats. A study at the University of Salerno, Italy, found that digestive enzymes significantly improved bloating, flatulence, and abdominal pain in patients with IBS.[13]

Taking one or two capsules at the beginning of each meal can ensure that foods are fully digested, decreasing the chance that partially digested food particles and proteins are damaging your gut wall or worse—sneaking through your tight junctions and into your bloodstream.[14]

---

key is to find a replacement for wheat flour. (Take note: I'm not saying it's a good idea to just eat gluten-free doughnuts. Sugary junk food is sugary junk food, gluten or no gluten!) Two flours that I like and recommend to my patients are coconut and almond flour.

Most people will do great with either of these flours, but for those with severe leaky gut, **coconut flour** is the best. I love the texture of coconut flour, which you can find in any natural grocery store. We enjoy making coconut flour blueberry muffins, coconut flour crepes, coconut flour chocolate chip cookies . . . you name it, you can make it with coconut flour.

Coconut flour is high in fiber, protein, and healthy fats. I also like that coconut flour scores low on the glycemic index and has more fiber and fewer carbohydrates than wheat flour. Made from ground and dried coconut meat, coconut flour isn't like the household "flour" you grew up with, but it sure is healthier. A study in the *Journal of Medicinal Food* showed that coconut flour's high nutrient density can help lower bad LDL cholesterol levels in those with raised cholesterol levels.[15]

If the texture of coconut flour isn't to your liking, you can try

GLUTEN HIDING IN PLAIN SIGHT

The amount of gluten found in wheat has doubled in recent years, thanks to those hybridized crops. Gluten is also added as a filler and binding agent to many processed food products, including:

- artificial coffee creamer
- bouillon cubes
- candy
- chewing gum
- snack chips
- cold cuts
- fish sticks
- flavored teas
- gravies
- ground spices
- hot dogs
- imitation seafood
- ketchup
- mayonnaise
- rice mixes
- salad dressing
- soy sauce
- tomato sauces
- vegetable cooking sprays

You won't find "gluten" on any of these food ingredient labels, but you will read head-scratching descriptions like:

- dextrin, malt, or maltodextrin
- gelatinized starch
- hydrolyzed plant protein (HPP)
- hydrolyzed vegetable protein (HVP)
- modified food starch
- monosodium glutamate (the infamous MSG)
- natural flavorings
- rice malt or rice syrup
- whey protein concentrate
- whey sodium caseinate

As we discussed in part 1, I believe gluten is a key reason for our nation's autoimmune crisis, with clear, documented links to diseases like celiac disease, type 1 diabetes, and Crohn's disease. Gluten has also been associated with more than fifty-five other diseases and is a major trigger for several thyroid conditions, including Hashimoto's disease. A study at the University of Turin in Italy demonstrated a strong link between celiac disease, caused by gluten, and the health of the thyroid.[16]

Even if you don't notice any obvious problems, consuming gluten puts your gut at risk for damage. So why eat it at all? I suggest steering clear of all gluten-containing foods.

almond flour. Sometimes I'll use a combination of the two. Almond flour is high in protein, fiber, and minerals and is best sprouted. Even though almond flour is healthy, I don't recommend consuming more than a quarter cup total in a sitting because almond flour can be hard to digest in large amounts. What both coconut flour and almond flour offer is great versatility in recipes with the bonus of healthy nutrients and filling fats.

When looking for gluten-free grains, **sprouted ancient grain flours (such as sprouted buckwheat, sorghum, amaranth, quinoa, or millet flour)** can also be a good option for those with mild to moderate leaky gut. **Sprouted corn, sprouted oat, and sprouted rice flour** are other possible substitutes for baking.

— Oil Outlaws —

Any time you're baking with coconut flour or almond flour, you're going to use some form of oil, right? But the oil of choice in many homes is canola oil or other vegetable oils, which are horrible for your health for two main reasons: 1) over 90 percent of canola oil and other vegetable oils, including corn oil and soybean oil, are produced from genetically modified plants; 2) vegetable oils are used in partially hydrogenated oils.

Partially hydrogenated oils are liquid fats that have been injected with hydrogen gas at high temperatures and under high pressure to make them solid at room temperature. This hydrogenation process produces a terrifying health villain: trans fats. Trans fats interfere with normal cell metabolism, and research shows that trans fats are hazardous for your heart because they lower the good HDL cholesterol, increase the bad LDL cholesterol, and increase triglycerides, a type of fat found in your blood. We need triglycerides for energy, but too many raise the risk of cardiovascular disease.

Hydrogenated fats have been linked to a *long* list of health conditions, including:

▶ atherosclerosis
▶ birth defects

- ▸ bone and tendon problems
- ▸ cancer
- ▸ diabetes
- ▸ digestive disorders
- ▸ heart disease
- ▸ immune system impairment
- ▸ increased cholesterol levels
- ▸ learning disabilities
- ▸ liver problems
- ▸ low birth weight
- ▸ obesity
- ▸ reduced growth
- ▸ sexual dysfunction
- ▸ skin reactions
- ▸ sterility
- ▸ vision reduction

Staggering, huh? We need to steer clear of these dangerous fats.

Another form of fat we need to approach with caution is omega-6 fatty acids, which are found in vegetable oils such as corn oil, safflower oil, sunflower oil, and soybean oil. When consumed in the wrong proportion, omega-6 fats cause inflammation of the intestinal lining, leading to leaky gut. These oils are base ingredients in nearly all processed foods, from baked goods to salad dressings. The solution is as simple as going to your pantry and tossing out the offending oils and replacing them with unrefined extra virgin coconut oil, ghee (clarified butter), olive oil, and flaxseed oil.

Extra virgin coconut oil is one of the healthiest and most versatile unprocessed oils in the world and remains stable when heated so you can cook with it. Today there are more than fifteen hundred studies proving the health benefits of coconut oil, including balancing hormones, eliminating candida, improving digestion and supporting metabolism, balancing blood lipids and sugar, and improving memory for those with Alzheimer's disease, among many others.

The vast majority (more than 85 percent) of the fats in coconut oil are medium-chain triglycerides. The medium-chain fatty acids (MCFAs) found in coconuts are easy for the body to burn as fuel for energy and have anticandida properties, in addition to other important traits.

Coconut oil contains three unique fatty acids that are responsible for its various health benefits: lauric, capric, and caprylic. These are some of the rarest substances found in nature and the reason why this oil is so beneficial.

Lauric acid has a particular structure that allows the body to absorb it easily. Once absorbed, lauric acid morphs into monolaurin, a chemical found in human breast milk. Monolaurin is known for its antiviral, antimicrobial, and antibacterial properties. For this and so many other reasons, coconut oil should be the go-to oil in the household, especially for cooking. You can be assured that coconut oil never shows signs of going rancid, even after a year at room temperature.

I use a lot of coconut oil in my baking recipes, but I'll use **ghee** when I want my baked items to have more of a buttery taste. Ghee is clarified butter—unsalted butter that is heated until the milk solidifies and rises to the top, which is then skimmed off and discarded. When all the milk solids and moisture are removed, ghee becomes more suitable for those with lactose intolerance. Ghee also contains high levels of alpha-linolenic acid (ALA) and conjugated linolenic acid (CLA), which help control blood clotting, build cell membranes in the brain, and reduce inflammation, helping soothe leaky gut. Ghee is also free of A1 beta-casein, so many people tolerate it better than conventional dairy products.

Olive oil should not be heated at any time because the healthy fats can oxidize, which makes it unsuitable for cooking. When used as the principal ingredient of salad dressing, however, olive oil is a fantastic form of fat, one that is a cornerstone of the Mediterranean diet (which features a high consumption of fruits, vegetables, whole grains, and legumes). In the past few decades, a large body of evidence has found healthy associations between the Mediterranean diet and mortality rates, incidence of coronary heart disease, and various types of cancer, according to a comprehensive study published in the journal *Clinical Interventions in Aging*.[17]

Finally, I want to mention **flaxseed oil**, which has anti-inflammatory properties and contains high levels of essential fatty acids (EFAs). Flaxseed oil can be used in smoothies or salad dressings but is consumed more often as a nutritional supplement or used as a healing balm than as a cooking oil. I often recommend it for those suffering from constipation, as flaxseed oil helps to lubricate the colon and soothe an inflamed gut. A review of studies by University of Maryland researchers showed that flaxseed oil and other omega-3 fatty acids may also be helpful in treating high cholesterol, heart disease, and cellular function.[18]

— Sugar Sabotage —

When it comes to foods with the potential to rip holes in your gut lining, sugar is one of the worst offenders. There's not much disagreement in the scientific and medical communities that sugar is a toxin of the highest rank, the sweetest poison of them all and lethal in many ways.

Sugar is found in nearly every man-made food, from breakfast cereal and yogurt to luncheon meat and wheat bread to ketchup, marinades, and salad dressings. Sugar is made from refined sugarcane and sugar beets in a process that creates the white crystals we all know so well while also removing the vitamins and minerals the plant fibers once possessed. The result is a pure, refined carbohydrate that has become the bane of modern society, responsible for causing huge spikes in insulin that promote fat storage. Over time, your insulin receptor sites can burn out, which leads to type 2 diabetes. Emerging research suggests that, much like the proven link with type 1 diabetes, leaky gut may also play a role in the type 2 diabetes epidemic worldwide.[19]

Eating too much sugar increases your risk of dying of heart disease, even if you aren't overweight. In a major study from the Harvard School of Public Health published in *JAMA Internal Medicine*, researchers looked at 15 years of data on over 40,000 people. After they accounted for the participants' age, sex, education level, physical activity, health eating index, and body mass index, they found that those participants who took in 25 percent or more of their daily calories as sugar were more than twice as likely to die from heart disease as those whose diets included less than 10 percent added sugar.[20]

According to the U.S. Department of Agriculture, the average American consumes 66 pounds of added sugar every year.[21] In comparison, we consume just one pound per year of mankind's oldest sweetener—**honey**.[22] Coming from the nectar of flowers through the efforts of busy bees toiling in the sunshine, honey contains a staggering number of antioxidants, minerals (including iron, zinc, potassium, calcium, phosphorus, magnesium, and selenium), and vitamins (vitamin B_6, thiamin, riboflavin, pathothenic acid, and niacin). Honey can also help to neutralize free radical activity in the body and act as a prebiotic to help feed and support our beneficial gut bacteria. One tablespoon of honey contains sixty-four calories, which is a little more than a tablespoon of refined sugar, but packs a nutritional bonanza in comparison.

But there's honey . . . and there's **raw honey**. Commercial honey is often heavily processed, so much so that 76 percent of honey products sold in U.S. grocery stores contains *zero* pollen and are devoid of other nutrients, making it really just another form of processed sugar.[23] The bee pollen in raw honey, however, contains natural microbes that help in modulating the immune response in the body. In addition, as we talked about in chapter 4, raw honey that is native to your region is best because it helps teach your gut bacteria how to build up an immune defense to local allergens. Consuming small, regular quantities of raw honey from your own county or region is a great delivery mechanism of microexposures of local dirt, helping you get more of those "old friends" back into your digestive system.

Aside from local honey, my favorite form of honey and one I've recommended to patients over the years is **manuka honey**. A unique form of honey harvested in New Zealand, manuka honey has tremendous antimicrobial properties that have been shown to improve symptoms of acid reflux by balancing out microbes in the stomach and intestines. According to New Zealand researchers, manuka honey reacts with the body's fluids to produce hydrogen peroxide, which creates an inhospitable environment for bad bacteria in the gut.[24] I recommend reducing your overall sugar intake from the American average of 126 grams of added sugar daily[25] to 20 to 40 grams and replace that added sugar with natural sweeteners such as manuka honey, dates, maple syrup, or—as I will talk about in the next section—stevia.

It's important to note that just as eating too much sugar swings the pendulum in the wrong direction, so does eating too much honey.

The wisest man who ever lived, King Solomon, once said, "Do you like honey? Don't eat too much, or it will make you sick!"[26]

— Artificial Deception —

We've all sat down in restaurants and noticed the small ceramic containers filled with blue, pink, and yellow packets of Equal, Sweet'N Low, and Splenda. We've all seen friends and family members reach for a packet to sweeten a cup of coffee or an iced tea. The promise of "zero calories" is a siren song that's proven to be irresistible to many dieters.

Those blue, pink, and yellow packets contain the artificial sweeteners aspartame, saccharin, and sucralose, respectively. They're toxic and dangerous and have been a source of controversy since the first artificial sweetener, saccharin, was discovered in 1879 at Johns Hopkins University. Saccharin, aspartame, and sucralose generally came to market in the 1960s and 1970s, giving researchers enough time—in my mind—to clarify any hazardous side effects. But these artificial sweeteners are still on the market, causing symptoms that range from headaches and migraines to even serious conditions like cardiovascular disease and type 2 diabetes, according to a 2013 study in *Trends in Endocrinology and Metabolism*.[27]

And then there's the risk of cancer, which makes artificial sweeteners a top gut grenade. Studies that have purported to show a link between cancer and an artificial sweetener like aspartame—sold under the brand names NutraSweet and Equal and found in beverages such as Diet Coke, Diet Pepsi, and Sugar Free Kool-Aid—have erupted into bitter controversy over the years.

While FDA studies have "ruled out" the cancer risk for nonnutritive sweeteners like aspartame, I have to wonder about the twenty-four-ounces-a-day average for drinkers of diet soda. It's been my experience that those who drink diet soda develop near-addiction responses, with some people drinking as many as six to twelve cans a day. What's all that chemical-laden slush doing to their gut and immune system?

In 2015, PepsiCo—the makers of Diet Pepsi, Caffeine Free Diet

Pepsi, and Wild Cherry Diet Pepsi—announced that the company had stopped sweetening their diet sodas with aspartame, the most problematic of the artificial sweeteners, and replaced this artificial sweetener with sucralose, better known as Splenda. Unfortunately, that isn't much of an improvement.

A study published in the journal *Environmental Toxicology* found sucralose has a more detrimental effect on gut bacteria than other artificial sweeteners because 65 to 95 percent of sucralose makes it all the way through the digestive tract and is excreted through feces unchanged.[28] Essentially, the body cannot digest sucralose, so this artificial sweetener travels through the GI tract causing damage as it goes—killing probiotics and harming the intestinal wall. Researchers at Duke University Medical Center also discovered that Splenda not only significantly reduces beneficial bacteria in the gut; this artificial sweetener

NOT-SO-SWEET SURPRISE

You don't have to pop open a can of diet soda for artificial sweeteners to leave a bad taste in your mouth. You may be surprised to learn that artificial sweeteners are included in many prepared foods, beverages, and even medications, including:

▶ toothpaste and mouthwash
▶ children's chewable vitamins
▶ chewing gum
▶ no-calorie "fitness" waters
▶ fizzy soft drinks
▶ flavored teas
▶ mixers for alcoholic beverages
▶ salad dressings
▶ frozen yogurt and other frozen desserts
▶ yogurt
▶ breakfast cereals
▶ processed snack foods
▶ "lite" or diet fruit juices and beverages
▶ processed meats

also increases your fecal pH, which decreases the amount of nutrients you can absorb.[29]

PepsiCo's move away from aspartame is a reaction to recent marketplace trends: people are simply not buying Diet Pepsi. Sales of this popular diet drink have plummeted 35 percent in the last ten years because a cultural tipping point has been reached about the dangers of this particular artificial sweetener. But, unfortunately, PepsiCo's decision to add sucralose doesn't improve matters. Although billed as a natural sugar substitute six hundred times sweeter than sugar, sucralose is a chlorinated sucrose derivative. Sucralose was actually discovered in a lab during development of a new insecticide compound and was never intended to be consumed by humans—but here we are.

If you're expecting artificial sweeteners to help you lose weight, think again. Purdue University researchers learned that sugar substitutes can interfere with the body's natural ability to count calories based on a food's sweetness. The Multi-Ethnic Study of Atherosclerosis (MESA), which included more than six thousand individuals, found that daily consumption of diet soda increased the risk for increased waist circumference and increased the chance of developing type 2 diabetes by 67 percent.[30]

So, what do you do when you order a tea in a restaurant but are determined not to reach for the packets of pure cane sugar or an artificial sweetener? Reach into your purse or pocket for a two-ounce bottle or powder packets of **stevia**, a sugar substitute derived from the stevia plant that grows in Paraguay and Brazil, where the indigenous people have used leaves from the stevia bush to add sweetness to their food for centuries. Stevia has no calories and is two hundred times sweeter than sugar in the same concentration—and it doesn't raise blood sugar levels. Stevia, however, does have a bitter aftertaste for some, so this sweetener isn't the perfect solution. Brands like SweetLeaf Stevia tend to be less bitter and have a more desirable aftertaste.

Not all stevia products are created equal. The best option is **green leaf stevia**, which is "only" thirty to forty times sweeter than sugar and has a sweeter, slightly less bitter taste. Stevia extracts are acceptable, but stay away from processed versions like Truvia, which really isn't stevia at all.

If the slightly bitter aftertaste of stevia is something you can't get used to, raw honey can sweeten any drink.

— Gut Protectors: Healing Foods —

You can begin to heal your gut today with these top healing foods. You'll learn more about each one of these foods as we continue through part 2. Start with one serving of each, and add as your system tolerates it. (And if you're having significant immune system issues, start off any fermented foods with a small amount, say half a teaspoon, to test your response.)

- ▸ **Bone broth** can transform your health. Both bone broth and collagen protein powder contain amino acids such as proline, glycine, and glutamine that help repair the gut lining. Along with gut-sealing collagen, bone broth is full of minerals—calcium, magnesium, phosphorus, silicon, sulfur— in forms that your body can easily absorb.
- ▸ **Fermented vegetables** enhance nutrients by making them more easily absorbed by the body, while restoring vital bacteria to your gut.
- ▸ **Coconut products** are high in lauric acid, which kills pathogens such as bacteria and fungi.
- ▸ **Fermented dairy** (yogurt and kefir) provide you with healthy bacteria to start rebalancing your gut flora.
- ▸ **Cooked vegetables** are easier to digest than raw and are packed with vitamins, minerals, and antioxidants.
- ▸ **Organic meat** products such as wild-caught fish and grass-fed beef are high in omega-3 fats and protein, which help reduce inflammation and rebuild healthy cells.

We've covered some of the foods that are the most dangerous for our gut, and talked about a few great alternatives. These food swaps are so delicious and nourishing you will not find yourself missing your old gut grenades for one second.

Next, let's talk about the second gut factor: our addiction to oversanitation.

6

A Sanitized Society

We are engaged in an ongoing battle for our microbiome, and our guts are ground zero. Unfortunately, this is a battle we have brought upon ourselves. Since the time of Pasteur, we've been trying to eradicate bacteria from every corner of our lives—from our increasing reliance on prescription and over-the-counter medications, to antibiotic use in conventional farming, to antibacterial agents mixed into everything from kitchen cleaners to gym mats and pencils. In an innocent attempt to keep ourselves safe from harm and "kill 99 percent of bacteria on contact," as the ads say, all of these modern innovations have contributed to the demise of our precious beneficial bacteria.

Luckily we don't have to look far to find inspiration on how to reverse course—it's really only in the past fifty to one hundred years that we've become fixated on eradicating bacteria, germs, and dirt. Once we make a conscious effort to welcome back dirt, we can also welcome back our beneficial microbes. Thankfully, reintegrating microbes into our lives requires much less work than the never-ending futility of trying to get rid of them!

— Helping Bad Bugs Bite the Dust —

I grew up in a home where my mother was constantly nagging us to wash our hands with antibacterial soap and reminding us not to get dirty when we went outside to play. In the kitchen, she regularly scrubbed down our counter with household bleach. The sink was so shiny that it sparkled, and our floors were spotless. Many of the moms I meet in my practice have the same exacting standards for their homes. After all, they want to protect their families' health.

But staying healthy involves good sanitation, not oversanitation. One animal study published in *Science* in 2012 demonstrated the harm that can result from living in a too-sterile environment. Researchers observed two groups of mice: the first group was bred with "germ-free" immune systems that lacked gut bacteria; the second group was given normal, healthy exposure to good and bad bacteria. When they were tested, the germ-free mice were found to have much higher levels of inflammation in their colon and lungs than the mice with normal germ exposure (who had healthy immune responses). The germ-free mice had also developed symptoms similar to ulcerative colitis and asthma. But the good news is, once the germ-free mice were exposed to normal amounts of bacteria two weeks after birth, their immune system response balanced out, and the animals healed from their inflammatory conditions.[1]

As studies like this demonstrate, strengthening your inner soil is essential to maintaining gut health and preventing inflammation. Because when your microbiome takes a hit early in life, the effects can be long-lasting—and severe. My patient Evan is living proof of that.

When I was a couple of years into my practice in Nashville, a pastor of a local church approached me with a concerned look on his face. "Dr. Josh, we've got this young guy in our congregation who's really sick," the pastor explained. "He was studying music at Belmont University, but he had to drop out because of severe digestive problems. What's happened is really a shame because he's an amazing pianist, but he's in such bad shape that he can't play in public any longer."

And that's how I came to know Evan, a nineteen-year-old student who'd been diagnosed with ulcerative colitis and Crohn's disease—both serious digestive disorders. I looked at his diet. It wasn't great. Before his health was compromised, he followed the typical college student burger-and-fries routine. But two years into his studies, he came down with painful diarrhea, rectal bleeding, and severe abdominal cramps, and his physician directed him to eat salads and fruit.

Big mistake.

The raw foods promoted inflammation in Evan's gut and made matters far worse for him. When you have inflammatory bowel disease (IBD), you don't want to eat raw foods, because the gut lining becomes so damaged that it can't handle a lot of fiber.

I asked Evan several more questions and learned that he had a history of prescription antibiotic use and took several other medications to treat immune-related issues. Since he'd been taking antibiotics since his early teen years, I knew he had developed a severe probiotic deficiency and had leaky gut syndrome. Evan was also taking prednisone, a corticosteroid prescription drug with immunosuppressant qualities—yet another hit to his microbiome.

I told Evan that I would ask him to follow a simple diet for two weeks where he could eat only three things: goat's milk kefir, bone broth, and cooked vegetables. I also asked him to take some probiotics derived from soil-based organisms twice a day. Evan had never heard of bone broth or kefir, so I gave him directions to the nearest Whole Foods and farmer's markets and sent him on his way. "Make sure to look for the veggies that have the most dirt on them," I reminded him on his way out.

Evan was a great patient. He took all his probiotics, drank his goat's milk kefir for breakfast and as an afternoon snack, and had bone broth with cooked vegetables for lunch and dinner. After two weeks on my diet, he felt so much better that his gastroenterologist removed the port that drained infections from his intestines. We then added other easy-to-digest foods, including organic meat, warm smoothies, coconut oil, avocados, and fruit.

Three months later, a healthy Evan reenrolled at Belmont and resumed his pursuit of a career in music.

Six months after Evan's initial consultation, I was invited to a concert at Belmont University where he was the solo pianist. His performance was inspiring, and my applause wasn't just for his gift as a musical prodigy—I was so proud of his commitment to making a health comeback.

I love success stories like Evan's, but his· health recovery is representative of how years of trying to blast his bad bacteria had also wiped out a large volume of good bacteria in his gut. Damaging that ideal 85-to-15 ratio, he'd triggered the leaky gut cycle that eventually led to his autoimmune condition. His microbiome was tapped out, almost to the point of bacterial bankruptcy—but his rapid infusion of probiotics came to the rescue, building up his reserves once more.

— Microexposures Help the Most —

Our task is to find ways to bring dirt back into our lives in a way that allows us to stay clean enough to guard against colds and flu, but also get dirty enough to enable our good microbes to do their work. The best, safest, and easiest way to do that is with those daily microexposures of dirt. One easy microexposure you can incorporate immediately is to consume more locally grown foods. The microbes in your local

WHAT ABOUT WASHING HANDS?

In our discussion of welcoming dirt back into our lives, I don't want to discount the importance of washing your hands. Unfortunately, our hands easily pick up large amounts of *bad* germs and bacteria as we go about our day. It is still important to wash your hands after you've touched public surfaces with an excess of potentially harmful microbes, such as those found in public restrooms.

When it comes to washing hands, I recommend warm water and essential oils like tea tree oil that have mild antimicrobial qualities. A lot of antibacterial soaps on the market today contain harsh chemicals like triclosan, which kill off the good bacteria as well as the bad. Triclosan (which is found in soaps, shampoos, sanitizers, and many other personal care products) has been shown to damage the liver and kidneys and cause cancer. I strongly suggest skipping the antibacterial hand washes and washing your hands with warm water and antimicrobial essential oils like orange, melaleuca, or rosemary oil. If you must buy hand soap, look for all-natural brands (such as Dr. Bonner's Pure Castile Soaps) that are free of chemical fragrances and additives such as retinyl acetate.

soil will help you better digest the foods grown in it, while also training your immune system to have a more customized response to the pathogens in your surrounding area.

The surest route to good health is to get these microbes in small doses over time—a little bit every day. Let's consider a few ways to incorporate these microexposures into our lives.

— Dirt on Our Bodies —

Americans are obsessed with personal hygiene. We take a lot of showers—nearly one a day, which is more than the British, Japanese, and Chinese.[2] Dr. Julia Segre, head of the Human Microbiome Project, has noted previous studies showing that showering can disrupt the balance of microorganisms on the skin, disbanding them into the air and surrounding cells. Daily showers may damage the outermost protective layer of the skin and disrupt the delicate balance maintained by the bacterial ecosystem that inhabits our skin. Indeed, many disruptive skin conditions, such as eczema and psoriasis, are autoimmune conditions with strong links to leaky gut.

One ammonia-oxidizing bacterium (AOB), called *Nitrosomonas eutropha*, is often found in dirt and untreated water, but was once also present in our skin bacteria, before we started washing it away. Scientists believe this bacteria actually kept us clean and fresh-smelling, boosted our immune system, and tamped down inflammation, all by feeding on the ammonia in our sweat and converting it into nitrite and nitric oxide.[3] While Americans no longer have AOB on their skin, scientists have found it on the skin of the Yanomami people.

The market is just starting to pick up on the potential for this alternative method of probiotic microexposures. (An interesting brand that's just been introduced is the Mother Dirt's AO+ line of soap, shampoo, and mist, which features AOB that's claimed to help keep you clean without washing.) If you can't bring yourself to go whole hog with an AOB-based product, I suggest you let your own body do the work of repopulating your skin by showering only on days you work out and just using **water without soap and shampoo** a few days a week. If you don't work out daily, then showering every other day is sufficient.

One of the ways I have helped my patients stay clean and use proper sanitation—yet not go overboard—is by asking them to try essential oils, another amazing way to use nature's healing compounds to replace the chemicals that have been poisoning our microbiome. Essential oils are one of our very oldest, most versatile, and most beneficial ways of "eating dirt."

Oils Through the Ages

For more than five thousand years, cultures around the world have extracted organic compounds from plants for their use in healing and beauty rituals. Egyptians in the days of Pharaoh made extensive use of essential oils in medicine and burial practices. When King Tut's tomb was opened in 1923, archaeologists discovered fifty alabaster jars filled with essential oils. Cleopatra, considered the most beautiful woman in the world, traveled from Egypt to the Dead Sea, where the waters naturally contained clay and minerals that were absorbed by her skin—the world's first clay mask! Cleopatra used essential oils like rose, frankincense, cypress, neroli, and myrrh, and was said to be "clouded in a scent of mystery." In the Bible, essential oils were used by Moses and other biblical figures to anoint kings; priests also used essential oils for healing. In fact, in the Book of Exodus, Moses was given a specific formula directly by God:

> Then the Lord said to Moses, "Take the following fine spices: 500 shekels [around 12 pounds] of liquid myrrh, half as much [around six pounds] of fragrant cinnamon, 250 shekels [around six pounds] of fragrant calamus, 500 shekels [around 12 pounds] of cassia—all according to the sanctuary shekel—and a hin [around a gallon] of olive oil. Make these into a sacred anointing oil, a fragrant blend, the work of a perfumer. It will be the sacred anointing oil."
> —Exodus 30:22–25 (NIV)

This formula was followed to make the holy anointing oil poured onto the heads of leaders or those suffering from a health ailment. In other words, this anointing oil wasn't just used for spiritual rituals, but was known to have healing properties.

Following the birth of Christ, the biblical story says, wise men from the Far East gave the infant king gifts of gold to honor his royalty, frankincense as a perfume, and myrrh for anointing oil. Frankincense oil was often rubbed on children to reduce swelling because of its anti-inflammatory qualities as well as immune protection. Myrrh oil was known as a natural antiseptic and could have been put on the infant Jesus' umbilical cord area as well as been applied to his mother, Mary, since myrrh oil helps heal tissues and balance hormones. Essential oils are referenced 264 times in the Bible, and 33 different types of oils are mentioned.

The father of medicine himself, the physician Hippocrates, utilized aromatherapy in Ancient Greece to enhance massage techniques. And practitioners of medicine in China and India have also employed herbal remedies and embraced essential oils for millennia.

Clearly, all major civilizations throughout history have relied upon essential oils' healing properties. But not only has history proven the benefits of essential oils, science has as well. Over 10,000 studies have been published on the therapeutic value of essential oils. Indeed, over 1,200 alone have looked at the properties of peppermint oil, a fact that's of particular interest because of peppermint's traditional use (now scientifically validated) as a tonic to soothe and heal the gut.

Using Essential Oils Safely and Effectively

When starting an essential oils routine, it's important to keep in mind that not all essential oils are created equal. In fact, many are worthless and some are even potentially toxic. There are four grades of essential oils:

1. **Synthetic and altered oils.** These oils are created in laboratories and are considered the lowest grades of oil.
2. **Natural and "pure" oils.** Although of better quality, these oils are overly processed, so they lose healing compounds. Natural oils are the most commonly sold type of essential oils.
3. **Therapeutic-grade essential oils.** These medicinal oils have been steam-distilled with healing compounds. The only

drawback about these oils is that they may be derived from plants and herbs that have been grown using pesticides.

4. **Certified organic therapeutic-grade essential oils.** These are the highest grade of essential oils from certified organic sources with the greatest healing properties.

How are these high-quality essential oils created? First, plants are organically grown and tended in accordance with their natural life cycle (as opposed to the artificially accelerated life cycle of industrial agriculture), so they're harvested when their healing compounds are most available. Next, their oils are extracted using steam distillation, CO_2 extraction, or cold-pressed methods without using chemicals. Finally, the oils are transferred to dark glass bottles for storage, which protects the fragile oils from oxidation and sunlight.

There are three main ways to access the healing power of essential oils:

1. A **topical application** penetrates the skin and passes into the bloodstream. Using essential oils in body products, like moisturizers and soaps, is an easy way to get in more daily microdoses of dirt. (Check out chapter 17 for DIY recipes you can make at home.)

2. Essential oils can be **aromatically absorbed** into the bloodstream when inhaled from a diffuser. A large number of blood vessels in the lungs absorb the oils and then circulate them throughout the body. You can diffuse lavender to reduce stress, tea tree oil (also known as melaleuca) to cleanse the air, wild orange to improve mood, frankincense to liven the spirits, and peppermint to improve focus and energy. (See chapter 10 for more condition-specific suggestions.)

3. The **ingestion** of essential oils can be a powerful form of medicine, but it must be noted that before using oils internally, you should either be working with a natural health care practitioner or talk to your doctor. Some essential oils are beneficial for internal use, but not all are safe for inges-

tion. Usually adding one to two drops of an essential oil into a cup of water is plenty. Oils like peppermint, lemon, and frankincense, when added to water, have considerable internal benefits. Certain oils such as oregano and clove can be used internally but only in very small amounts and for no longer than one week.

BONUS: If you want to learn more about how to use essential oils and their benefits you can download my free essential oil book here: www.draxe .com/essential-oils-book-bonus

---

— Dirt in Our Mouths —

In today's world, we have to be proactive to seek out foods that still contain their natural quantities of beneficial bacteria and enzymes. The majority of the foods we consume have been pasteurized (heated between 161 and 280 degrees), irradiated (passed through radiation), or sprayed with pesticides—all of which damage beneficial organisms in our gut. Even when we do our best to seek out foods with beneficial microbes, we might still lose them when we run them under the tap to wash them. Varying levels of chlorine are found in the municipal water we wash our food in (and drink and bathe in) and chlorine has been shown to destroy good microbes on your skin and in your digestive tract. Research published in the *British Medical Journal* has also found that the fluoride in tap water damages the lining of the intestines, causing leaky gut and destroying beneficial bacteria.[4]

The stakes are certainly high. Here are a few more ways we can strengthen our inner soil and build up the microbiome.

SBOs, or Soil-Based Organisms

I call SBOs the king of probiotics. When these tiny microorganisms enter our bodies, they support gut health and immune response, and help us live long, healthy lives. In the plant world, soil-based organisms protect vegetation from disease and help plants grow to their fullest potential. Without the protection of SBOs—plant life's first line of defense—healthy vegetation becomes susceptible to unfriendly bacteria like fungi, yeasts, molds, parasites, and other pathogens in the dirt.

When we lived in an agrarian society, we had plenty of opportunities to get our hands dirty and come into contact with these helpful organisms. In 1900, half of the U.S. labor force were farmers. In just 115 years, that number has shrunk to just 2 percent—and 60 percent of today's hardworking farmers farm only part time. Very few of us get dirty working the soil or being around a dusty farming operation.

Since most people are living and working in dirt-free urban settings or suburbs, it's vital to make sure we actively seek out contact with SBOs. Unfortunately, most of our food supply does not contain dietary SBOs, with the exception of food from farmer's markets, where we can purchase fresh fruits and vegetables still coated with soil from the ground. This is where nutritional supplementation containing soil-based organisms steps into the gap.

Inside your gut, SBOs devote themselves to killing off the harmful bacteria that would otherwise make you sick. Every time you eat and send food to the digestive tract, they pull nutrients out of your food and make your entire digestive system work the way it should by breaking down proteins, carbohydrates, and nutrients into smaller pieces so they can be completely absorbed into the bloodstream and used by the body.

You can find hundreds of different species of SBOs in nature, but the best strains come from the *Bacillus* family. The first is *Bacillus subtilis*, an endospore probiotic that is heat resistant. *Bacillus subtilis* elicits a potent immune response, supports the healing of the gut lining, and suppresses the growth of bad bacteria like salmonella and other pathogens. This bacterium doesn't normally live in the human gastrointestinal tract, nor is it found in common foods, so you have to take it in supplement form.

The other strain is *Bacillus coagulans*, also an endospore probiotic that is heat resistant. This strain improves nutrient absorption. Upon activation of spore formation in the acidic environment of the stomach,

Bacillus coagulans can germinate and proliferate in the intestines and produce lactic acid, critical factors in the effectiveness of this probiotic. *Bacillus coagulans* has been shown to reduce inflammation and symptoms of arthritis, according to a study in the journal *BMC Complementary and Alternative Medicine.*[5]

If and when you seek out a nutritional supplement with SBOs, be sure to look for *Bacillus subtilis* and *Bacillus coagulans* on the product label.

Medicinal Mushrooms

In forested areas, mycelia—the parts of the mushroom that grow below the ground rather than the fruiting body on top—have been shown to detoxify the earth by breaking down plant and animal debris and turning that material into rich topsoil. Many are unaware that the most beneficial part of the mushroom is the mycelia.

When consumed by humans, mushroom mycelia offer many wonderful benefits that include:

- helping balance microbes in the microbiome
- supplying beneficial microbes with prebiotics, to keep them well fed
- effectively boosting the immune system
- detoxifying chemicals and heavy metals
- inhibiting pathological immune functions in autoimmune disorders
- reducing histamine release, which is associated with autoimmune disorders
- destroying tumors and cancer cells
- helping fight viruses and candida
- acting as an adaptogen to balance cortisol levels and other stress hormones

Many types of mushroom mycelia exist in nature, but five of the most powerful are cordyceps, reishi, shiitake, lion's mane, and turkey tail. All of these mushrooms have a history of medicinal use in ancient Chinese medicine that dates back thousands of years, and have immune-enhancing properties currently being studied around the world for their promise in fighting cancer. Let's take a closer look at each of these five mushrooms and how they can improve your health:

▶ **Cordyceps mushrooms,** known for their nutritive and tonic quali-ties, are found in the high altitudes of the Himalaya mountains and have been traditionally cooked into soups in Asia for centuries. Multiple studies in China have found that cordyceps shrinks tumors and prolongs the lifespan of mice. An Indian study published in the *Journal of Ethnopharmacology* showed that laboratory mice had a 73 percent increase in overall exercise endurance after supple-menting with cordyceps.[6] It's also been reported that cordyceps is especially helpful for treating chronic coughs, asthma, and other bronchial conditions.

▶ **Reishi,** an herbal mushroom, grows on decaying tree stumps across East Asia and North America. Hailed as the "mushroom of immor-tality," reishi's antioxidant actions are of keen interest to cancer researchers, including those at Memorial Sloan Kettering Cancer Center, who've noted that reishi mushrooms stimulate cells in the immune system. A 2013 study published in *PLOS One* studied the antitumor effects of reishi against breast cancer. After thirteen weeks of exposure to reishi, the tumors shrank by 50 percent. The researchers concluded that the reishi worked by improving cel-lular communication and reducing inflammation, which would be beneficial in fighting many types of cancers.[7] A study in the *Pro-ceedings of the National Academy of Sciences* also found that a type of carbohydrate molecule found in reishi mushrooms can induce antibodies to identify and destroy antigens associated with tumors or cancer cells.[8]

▶ **Shiitake** mushrooms are readily found in natural foods stores and widely served in Asian restaurants. Known as the "elixir of life" for centuries, shiitake has been investigated for its anticancer and immune-boosting properties. Shiitake is rich in selenium, an anti-oxidant, as well as vitamins A, C, D, and E. Shiitake mushrooms may also lower blood pressure for those with hypertension, lower cholesterol, increase libido, and stimulate antiviral effects in the body.

▶ **Lion's mane mushrooms** aren't anything like the classic cap-and-stem button varieties of mushrooms that shoppers are used to purchasing in the produce section. A review of mushrooms' anti-cancer properties published in the medical journal *3 Biotech* noted lion's mane's antitumor and immunomodulatory effects and found that extracts of the mushroom reduced tumor weights by almost 40 percent.[9]

Lion's mane mushrooms and their cascading tendrils have long been used in ancient Chinese medicine for the way they boost the immune and digestive systems. A 2013 study published in the journal *Evidence-Based Complementary and Alternative Medicine* found that lion's mane reduced intestinal inflamma-tion and protected the stomach from further damage by gastric ulcers.[10] Other research has also proven that lion's mane may help repair damaged nerves, improve memory, and stimulate the production of antioxidants like superoxide dismutase (SOD) and glutathione.

These mushrooms are found in hardwood forests throughout the world, but mainly in Asia and parts of Europe and North America. Lion's mane mushrooms intended for cooking are still making their way into more and more gourmet stores but are already widely available as an extract in nutritional supplements.

▶ **Turkey tail mushroom** is also known by its botanical name, *Trametes versicolor*. Readily found in the woods in nearly every state in the United States, the colorful stripes and banding pattern of this beguiling mushroom look like the tail of a strutting turkey. Most of the bands are dark to light brown in color, but other col-ors come into play, such as light green, orange, and purple, as the name "versicolor" suggests.

Paul Stamets, an internationally respected expert on mushrooms, claims turkey tail mushrooms can "heal the world" because of their power to both cleanse the soil of heavy metals and toxins and help heal humans' inner soil. According to Stamets, mushroom mycelia break down and detoxify the body of heavy metals, such as lead

GETTING YOUR MUSHROOMS IN A CAPSULE

Mushrooms have tremendous natural abilities to fight dangerous bacteria and viruses. According to a 2005 report published in the *Journal of Evidence-Based Complementary and Alternative Medicine*, mushrooms contain compounds and complex substances that include antimicrobial, antiviral, antitumor, antiallergic, immunomodulating, anti-inflammatory, heart-protecting, blood-sugar-lowering, and liver-protecting properties.[12] In fact, mushrooms need to have those strong antibacterial and antifungal compounds just to survive in their own natural environment, which is why it's not surprising that these beneficial compounds can be isolated from many mushrooms and used to protect human cells. That feature is fantastic news for many of my patients who simply cannot stand the taste or texture of mushrooms. If this sounds like you, supplements can help you access these tremendous healing powers without having to address the sensory issues of actually *eating* them. Look for mushrooms that have been proven to help modulate and build immunity, such as lion's mane, shiitake, cordyceps, reishi, and turkey tail.

and mercury, and remove industrial toxins from the soil, including pesticides and chlorine.

Stamets partnered with the National Institutes of Health (NIH) to study the use of turkey tail mushrooms as an adjunct therapy to radiation in breast cancer patients to support immune levels. His research showed that NK cells ("natural killer," helpful immune cells) increased tremendously in just six weeks, a demonstration of the cancer-fighting properties.[11]

Blue-Green Algae

An explanation is in order: blue-green algae are not just algae but also a form of bacteria that has an unusual blue-green coloration, hence its name. Nutrient-rich bodies of water, such as ocean bays and large freshwater lakes, support the rapid growth of blue-green algae. When high concentrations occur, the blue-green algae "bloom" and color the water in a distinctive bluish color.

Blue-green algae has long been one of the most nutrient-dense foods on the planet—and this includes its prebiotic power to feed the beneficial microbes in the gut. The Aztecs harvested blue-green algae from Lake Texcoco in central Mexico, and African tribespeople living on Lake Chad in west-central Africa discovered the health advantages of a dried-out form of blue-green algae centuries ago. These days, Hawaii is a premier source for blue-green algae.

One popular type of blue-green algae is spirulina, which is known for its high concentration of iron, B_{12}, calcium, niacin, potassium, magnesium, beta-carotene, and several B vitamins. NASA astronauts used this nutrient as a nutritional supplement on space missions. I've found spirulina to be an awesome addition to smoothies because of its intense flavor and powerful nutrition profile.

To date, there are nearly twelve hundred peer-reviewed scientific articles evaluating blue-green algae and spirulina, with seventy peer-reviewed articles examining spirulina's ability to affect cancer cells. According to the University of Maryland Medical Center, animal and test-tube studies suggest that "spirulina increases the production of antibodies, infection-fighting proteins, and other cells that improve immunity and help fight off infection and chronic illness such as cancer."[13] The Memorial Sloan Kettering Cancer Center notes that blue-green algae may protect against DNA mutations and increase levels of NK cells in humans.[14]

Spirulina and its blue-green algae cousin chlorella not only enhance probiotics in the microbiome but also protect good bacteria in the gut from being killed off. Radiation, heavy metals (which come from high concentrations of arsenic in drinking water or mercury in fish), and toxins can destroy probiotics in the gut, but spirulina and chlorella protect the digestive tract against these depletions. Clinical studies published in the peer-reviewed journal *Environmental Health Perspectives* suggest that chlorella aids in detoxification of polychlorinated dioxins in humans and may also protect the body from radiation exposure.[15]

Both spirulina and chlorella have a concentrated balance of nutrients that help cleanse and detoxify the body. Chlorella's protein levels and combination of vitamins, minerals, and phytonutrients go one step beyond spirulina. When used in tandem, their powers are synergistic. Unfortunately, chlorella's tough exterior walls are difficult to digest.

When purchasing a chlorella supplement, make sure you buy "cracked cell wall chlorella," which is completely absorbable.

While chlorella holds an abundance of health benefits, I give the edge to spirulina because of its nutrition density. If you have sinus issues or are looking to speed up weight loss, spirulina can help in these areas, too. Spirulina benefits the body by reducing inflammation that leads to itching, nasal discharge, congestion, and sneezing. As for losing weight, the protein-rich nature of spirulina curbs hunger.

Spirulina is also effective in eliminating candida. In the United States, candida overgrowth—a yeast infection—has become a hallmark sign for many autoimmune diseases today, according to a paper published in *Clinical Microbiology Reviews*.[16] The shift toward diets rich in sugar and unnatural ingredients as well as an increase in antimicrobial resistance and antifungal drugs has created a significant rise in yeast infections. A study published in the *Journal de Mycrologie Médicale* showed that spirulina is an effective antimicrobial agent and that the immune-strengthening properties of spirulina help the body eliminate candida cells.[17]

Regardless of your health issue or goal, I recommend that you add a teaspoon of spirulina to your daily smoothie or take it in supplement form from a reputable brand.

Phages

I wouldn't be surprised if you've never heard of or seen the word "phage" before. Phage comes from the word "bacteriophage"; bacteriophages are good viruses that attack bacteria but not humans. Phages are one of the most abundant life forms on earth, readily found in water and soil.

Phage therapy is the use of beneficial viruses to combat pathogenic bacteria. This form of therapy was popular in the first half of the twentieth century, but fell into disfavor after the discovery of antibiotics in the 1940s. With the rise of antibiotic-resistant bacteria suddenly grabbing attention in the medical world, the therapeutic potential of phages is getting a second look. In 2014, the American Society of Microbiology (ASM) listed phage therapy as one of seven ways we can begin to combat antibiotic resistance.

Since phages are viruses, there's been a reluctance to use them to treat infections. But initial trials with laboratory animals have shown that phages can kill more than 99 percent of *E. coli* cells that contain specific antibiotic-resistant gene sequences.[18] A 2011 review in the journal *Bacteriophage* included many studies that suggested phages have been beneficial in treating ear and eye infections, burns, cystic fibrosis and other lung diseases, antibiotic-resistant MRSA infections, and more.[19]

Since phages are abundant in salt water, taking a dip in the ocean can be one of the best ways to "eat dirt" and allow the body to receive a wonderful mix of minerals and microbes. I've had patients with acne tell me that after swimming in the ocean for a prolonged time, their skin improved tremendously. If you're fortunate enough to live fairly close to a coastline, then going for a seawater swim is an incredibly healing activity. If you live too far from the beach, you can find phages in certain probiotic and microbiome-balancing supplements.

Yeast

Yeast is another misunderstood microbe. Just as there are good and bad bacteria and fungi, there are good and bad types of yeast.

Few are aware that the body naturally produces yeast in the mouth, digestive tract, rectum, and vagina. One of the best ways to strengthen your inner soil is to introduce more good yeast into the digestive tract. One of the best yeasts out there is *Saccharomyces boulardii*, a friendly yeast that restores natural flora in the large and small intestine and improves intestinal cell growth.

Saccharomyces boulardii, pronounced *SAK-a-roe-MYE-sees-boo-LAR-dee*, is known for supporting healthy digestion. The name comes from a French microbiologist named Henri Boulard, who traveled to Indochina in the 1920s, long before the land became known as Vietnam. Dr. Boulard was there to study why the locals were dying from a cholera epidemic, which was marked by severe diarrhea. During his research, he observed that those who survived drank a tea from litchi fruit skins to combat the dysentery.

Intrigued, Dr. Boulard studied litchi fruit tea and managed to isolate the yeast responsible for curing the locals' diarrhea. The yeast didn't have a name, so Dr. Boulard nominated himself and called it *Saccharo-myces boulardii.*

Medical studies over the intervening decades have confirmed what Vietnamese folklore has espoused for centuries: if you have severe diarrhea, *Saccharomyces boulardii* helps you recover (by destroying pathogenic bacteria in the bowels). This friendly yeast can also relieve bloating and gas as well as repair the mucous membranes lining the intestinal walls and strengthen immune function in the digestive tract.

Saccharomyces boulardii not only functions like a probiotic in the body, it's also an antidote to all types of diarrhea, whether triggered by antibiotic use, traveling, or simply long-standing, chronic diarrhea. *Saccharomyces boulardii* has proven to be effective in treating inflammatory bowel disease such as Crohn's disease. It's also been shown to increase enzyme effectiveness, have antitoxin and antimicrobial effects, and reduce inflammation.[20, 21, 22]

The yeast also helps eliminate acne. A German study published in *Fortschritte der Medizin* discovered that more than 80 percent of patients, in a double-blind study, saw their acne condition healed or considerably improved as compared to 26 percent in a placebo group.[23]

And finally, even though *Saccharomyces boulardii* is a yeast, it can destroy a pathogenic yeast like *Candida albicans.* Researchers have found that *Saccharomyces boulardii* reduces inflammation and crowds out bad bacteria and yeast, resulting in improved digestion and skin improvements among those with chronic candida infections.

Shilajit

Here's another nutritional powerhouse that needs a pronunciation guide. Shilajit—pronounced *shee-lah-JEET*—is a dense, mineral-rich soil found high in the Himalayan mountains bordering India and Nepal. Sherpas, renowned for guiding mountain climbers to the top of Mount Everest, make shilajit part of their diet.

Shilajit contains at least eighty trace minerals, including two of my favorites—humic acid and fulvic acid—that are commonly used as a soil supplement in agriculture. Many of these eighty minerals have practically disappeared from our bodies because modern-day practices like spraying pesticides and herbicides have depleted the nutritive qualities of our soil. Because of its high mineral and nutrient content, shilajit has been touted as nature's multimineral supplement. Sourced from the world's tallest mountain chain, shilajit is one of the best ways to "eat dirt" in a supplement form.

In India, shilajit is called the "destroyer of weakness" because of the way this thick, resinous, jet-black (or dark brown) dirt delivers energy and nutrients to cells at better-than-expected levels. According to a study published in the journal *Science of Total Environment*, an Indian research team found that the fulvic acid in shilajit stimulates energy metabolism and protects cell membranes from oxidation, which is a main cause of aging, cancer, and inflammatory disease.[24]

Bentonite Clay

And don't forget, one of the great ways to eat dirt is to literally *eat dirt*—as in, small bits of clay.

We talked about bentonite clay in chapter 4. In case you're wondering if I put into practice what I preach, the answer is yes. I actually gargle with bentonite clay every day! I still remember one of the first times I ate this particular kind of dirt, and I couldn't be more grateful for how it helped me.

It was shortly after I finished my medical studies, and I went on a mission trip to Uganda and Ethiopia with a group called Visiting Orphans. We dropped in on several local orphanages, where we did small building projects and hung out with the kids. I count this time as one of the richest experiences in my life.

One evening in Ethiopia, our hosts took us to a local restaurant where we were served a "hot pot" with an array of Ethiopian ingredients. You can imagine all the different spices in the sauce along with the unfamiliar meats and vegetables in this Ethiopian stew. Long story short, that "hot pot" wrecked my stomach.

Now, had I approached the eating of that stew in microexposures, of say a spoon or two a day for a week or two, my system might have adjusted and I might have been able to eat the full hot pot meal without incident. But getting the full dose at once overwhelmed my gut and gave my system a more shocking introduction to the local microbiome.

I had brought some soil-based probiotic supplements with me as well as a vial of bentonite clay. I started taking a teaspoon of clay three times a day in filtered water, along with the probiotics. I felt a world of relief right away and kept up this regimen until a week later when I boarded the long flight back to the United States. I don't know what would have happened to me if I hadn't brought that vial of bentonite clay with me.

I will concede that "eating clay" isn't easy the first time around because of its grittiness, but try putting a half teaspoon into water, mixing it up, and then drinking it right away. Or use it as a mouth-wash—gargling for thirty seconds and spitting out the clay, then rins-ing your mouth with clean water. Clay has many health benefits and can be a very efficient way to get a high dose of dirt at a single time! But don't overdo it, because eating too much clay can cause major constipation.

Bone Broth

For a long time in our culture, meat on the bone was seen as the lowest cut—the bones were just part of the carcass, to be discarded with the rest of the offal. With the exception of prime rib, most expensive cuts of meat tend to be those with the least contact with bone—boneless chicken breasts, filet mignon, pork tenderloin. But what we're learning now is that bones and surrounding ligaments and cartilage may actually be among the most nourishing, nutrient-rich parts of the animal. And what better way to get at those nutrients than in a warm bowl of bone broth.

All bone broths—beef, chicken, fish, lamb, and more—are staples in the traditional diets of every culture. That's because bone broths are nutrient-dense, easy to digest, and rich in flavor and boost healing. Bone broth or stock was a way our ancestors made use of every part of an animal. Bones and marrow, skin and feet, tendons and ligaments can be boiled and then simmered over a period of days. This simmering causes the bones and ligaments to release healing compounds like col-lagen, proline, glycine, and glutamine, compounds shown to improve rheumatoid arthritis, other joint conditions, and inflammatory bowel disease—all linked directly to leaky gut.[25] One animal study published in *Pathophysiology* found that proline-containing peptides found in bone broth restored the mucosal lining in animals with leaky gut.[26]

Researchers at the Weston A. Price Foundation found bone broths also contain minerals in forms that your body can easily absorb: calcium, magnesium, phosphorus, silicon, sulfur, and others. They also contain chondroitin sulfates and glucosamine, the compounds sold as pricey supplements to reduce inflammation, arthritis, and joint pain.[27]

A study of chicken broth conducted by the University of Nebraska Medical Center considered what it was in the soup that made it so beneficial for colds and flu. Researchers found that the amino acids produced when making chicken stock reduced inflammation in the respiratory system and improved digestion. Also, further research suggests it helps the immune system heal from conditions such as allergies and asthma.[28]

While the dietary collagens found in all bone broths are beneficial, some are more beneficial than others. Bovine collagen is highest in type 1 and 3 collagen, beneficial for skin, hair, and nails. Chicken collagen includes type 2, found in our cartilage, and is particularly beneficial for the gut and joints. Fish collagen is perhaps the most beneficial of all, because it helps your body produce its own collagen and efficiently raises your levels of type 1 collagen, found in 90 percent of the tissues in the body.

When you make your bone broth, be sure to cook it with meat and fat as well as bone, to dilute any heavy metals (such as lead) that may be concentrated in the bone, and use organic, free-range animals whenever possible. To help "heal and seal" the intestinal lining in leaky gut, I usually recommend people drink 1 to 2 cups of bone broth a day and take a collagen supplement with all three types (1, 2, and 3) included. Collagen powders can also be a great way to sneak protein into a gut-healing smoothie.

Create Your Own Garden

At the edge of major cities in Germany and Switzerland lie large plots of land called *Schrebergartens,* where city dwellers can rent a ten-by-twenty-foot patch of land and get their hands dirty on weekends tending to their vegetables and flower beds. Many *Schrebergartens* have miniature houses, mature fruit trees, and white picket fences.

The rent-a-garden concept has been exported to U.S. cities in a modest way, but hasn't really caught on to the degree it has in Europe. Most of us don't have the time, the expertise, or any land to grow our own food. Others simply don't want to get their hands dirty messing with a garden. But consider how many benefits you'd get from this one hobby:

- ▶ less expensive (free!) organic produce
- ▶ more time touching, smelling, and tasting dirt
- ▶ regular exposure to SBOs—right in your backyard
- ▶ greater connection to the rhythms of nature—growing seasons, changes in the soil, time outside in the sun
- ▶ greater exposure to local pollen
- ▶ pride of a job well done

Even if you decide not to plant a garden, be sure to spend plenty of time outside every day. And please don't chastise your preschooler for sampling the mud pies he made in the backyard. A little dirt won't kill him. Most likely, he's eating some dirt anyway. The Environmental Protection Agency reports that the average toddler (three and under) consumes one teaspoon of dirt per day, which increases microbe diversity. So if children want to play in the dirt or run around the backyard with their shoes off, let them.

Today, eating dirt—something that humans have done naturally for millennia—has become a challenge. We have less and less contact with the natural world. Our food is essentially sterilized before it makes it onto grocery store shelves. And advancements in agricultural science have left us with a legacy of environmental toxins and soil degradation.

At the same time, many other untested innovations—from personal care products to nonstick cookware—have also unleashed harmful chemicals in our world. In the next chapter we will discuss how many of our modern inventions have backfired when it comes to supporting our health. The good news is there are some simple, old-fashioned steps you can take to repopulate your microbiome and protect your gut.

7

The Price of Convenience

Many of the gut-damaging foods we talked about in chapter 6 were introduced into our food supply for two very simple reasons: convenience and profit.

Our hectic and on-the-go lifestyles have created an increased demand for convenient foods. And in turn, enterprising manufacturers have answered with foods that too commonly ignore health consequences in favor of higher profits.

Unfortunately, both of these factors have succeeded in driving us further away from the simple, straight-from-the-source foods that our bodies need to stay strong and deal with the demands of modern life. Convenience has become addictive. While we've become increasingly dependent on convenience foods, we've also incorporated additional "convenience" products that are harmful to our health. Today we are exposed to more environmental toxins on a daily basis than ever before in history. These toxins—present in our food supply, our environment, and even our homes—threaten our health in many alarming ways. Let's take a look at a few ways these everyday toxins infect our lives and our guts.

— Trading Dirt for Convenience —

A couple of years ago, Chelsea and I traveled to Florence, Italy, where we took a cooking class that included a shopping tour of the open-air San Lorenzo Market. There we watched local restaurateurs peruse, sniff, feel, and barter for the best produce, meat, and cheeses with the local *venditore*.

It was incredible to take in the sights and smells of the bustling stalls and watch the local chefs carefully inspect the San Marzano tomatoes, known as *pomodori* in Italian, or "golden apples," for their tremendous flavor and texture. One of the most important lessons taught in our class was that most great Italian meals start with a foundation of fresh tomato sauce.

We also discovered that Italians make just enough tomato sauce—and whatever else they're preparing—to get them through the meal they're serving. The reason: they don't have room for leftovers in their refrigerators, which are often the size of a fridge you'd find tucked inside a college dorm room in the States.

The small refrigerators and wonderful tomatoes in Italy reflect a culture that understands the connection between the dirt and the table, between food quality and quality of life. In many European countries, fresh foods are the norm, not the exception. Many have actually banned genetically modified crops from their food supply altogether. Their default produce is fresh from a local farm, covered in life-giving soil-based organisms, and bursting with vibrant antioxidants and flavor.

In contrast, when we purchase our foods from a conventional grocery store, we are likely eating produce or animal products shipped in from thousands of miles away, teeming with toxic levels of hormones, antibiotics, and pesticides that have become the norm in America's modern industrial agriculture. Because our food supply is organized around a profit motive rather than a public health perspective, every change has led us further and further from the dirt, and deeper and deeper into a toxic swamp.

— The Siren Call of the Fridge and Microwave —

Refrigerators and microwave ovens have changed the nutritional value and the composition of the foods we eat—and not for the better. Produce quickly loses its nutrient value following harvest. Researchers at Penn State found that spinach lost 47 percent of its folate and carotenoids after only four days at room temperature or eight days in a refrigerator. And a University of California, Davis, study showed that vegetables can lose between 15 and 77 percent of their vitamin C content within a week after being picked. Dozens of other nutrients are quickly lost during transport and storage of fresh fruits and vegetables, because they are so sensitive to air, light, and heat. There's a reason why we call produce *perishable*.

Like just about every American, I believed that once I put a bag of organic spinach in the drawer of my refrigerator, it should be fine for at least a week, maybe longer. But if that bag of organic spinach took five days to reach a distribution center and a couple of days to get stocked at a grocery store, and spent another day or two in the cold case before I picked it up and dropped it into my shopping cart, how many vital nutrients were lost forever?

— The Real Problem: Pesticides and GMOs in Food Supply —

When the U.S. Senate launched an investigation into the decreasing quality of our soil, this is what it reported: "The alarming fact is that foods—fruits, vegetables and grains—now being raised on millions of acres of land that no longer contain enough of certain needed nutrients, are starving us—no matter how much we eat of them."[1]

That report was published in 1936.

By 1999, the U.S. Department of Agriculture found that forty-three vegetables and fruits showed "reliable declines" in protein, calcium, phosphorus, iron, vitamin B_2, and vitamin C in the previous fifty years. Average calcium levels in twelve fresh vegetables (such as broccoli, cabbage, carrots, onions, watercress, and kale) dropped 27 percent. Vitamin C levels had dropped 30 percent.[2, 3] The difference is so dramatic that we would have to eat eight oranges to get the same amount of vitamin C as our grandparents got from eating just one.

Despite all of our advances in technology and agricultural practices, the health of our soil is only getting worse. Our soil today has 85 percent fewer minerals than it contained 100 years ago.[4] If our farmers don't actively replenish these lost nutrients, the mineral content of our food will continue to decline.

The main culprit is soil depletion. Aggressive agricultural methods have literally stripped the minerals and nutrients out of the soil. Rather than using tried-and-true methods for letting the soil rebuild itself, the industry has defaulted to fast-growing, pest-resistant production, making every generation of produce less nutritious than the last.[5]

All over the world, minerals and nutrients in our soil have been lost because of these farming practices. Some estimate that only forty-eight years of nutrient-rich topsoil remains.

In some ways, minerals are more essential to our health than vitamins. Our bodies can't manufacture minerals, so we must get them from our diet. The minerals in food are supplied by the soil where the produce was grown. Healthy soil also helps to supply specific vitamins, natural antibiotics, amino acids, and phytochemicals vital to our health. Some of our worst chronic illnesses stem from nutritional deficiencies: heart disease, stroke, diabetes, obesity, bone loss, high blood pressure, dementia, macular degeneration, and leaky gut. If we fail to change our farming practices now, history has shown us that the results will negatively affect generations to come. Historically, entire civilizations have died off when their topsoil was depleted of nutrients.[6]

Those San Marzano tomatoes we cooked with in Florence are considered by chefs to be among the best tomatoes in the world. Sweet and luscious, with a thicker skin and fewer seeds, the tomatoes in Italy tasted much better than commercially grown tomatoes in the United States.

Whether grown in the States or in neighboring Mexico, our conventional tomatoes are picked from the vine while they are still green and then allowed to ripen on their way to market. Plant geneticists have manipulated present-day tomatoes to have specific characteristics: they must turn red by the time they reach the store, they must remain firm, and their skin has to be durable enough to travel long distances. Taste? Nutrition? Not part of the criteria.

A study published in the journal *Science* reported that the same gene that makes our tomatoes uniformly red also stifles the genes that produce the sugar and aromas that make up a fragrant, nutritionally potent, and flavorful tomato.[7] James J. Giovannoni of the U.S. Department of Agriculture Research Service, the author of the *Science* study, called this decades-long development of the modern-day tomato a "story of unintended consequences." The $300 billion agriculture industry is focused on getting your tomatoes and your produce from the farm to your shopping cart in the most efficient and profitable way possible. While consumers benefit from lower prices, we get what we pay for: bland and watery tomatoes, fruits and vegetables that lack the nutritional punch they should have.

Pesticides, herbicides, and fungicides, readily used by U.S. farmers to ward off insects and pests, leave behind a toxic chemical residue on produce that, when eaten, taxes the liver and the digestive system. One 2014 study published in *PLoS One* found that animals exposed to the farming pesticide chlorpyrifos experienced significant tight junction changes in their gut lining, and bacteria was found to have leaked through and migrated to the spleen.[8] From a clinical perspective, if the spleen is damaged by these pesticides, it can result in a downward spiral of negative health consequences from yeast overgrowth to blood issues such as anemia. The results of this study also suggested that concentrations of organophosphate pesticide at this level can be absorbed from food directly into the bloodstream. If these effects are so clearly seen among farm animals, what happens to us when we eat those same grains or vegetables—or even the farm animals themselves?

In late 2015, the EPA issued a proposal to ban pesticides like chlorpyrifos from farming practices due to the negative health consequences it produces. Unfortunately, as of this writing, it remains in use.[9]

— Just Say NO to GMO —

GMO foods are *another* modern development that have taken over Big Agriculture and are harmful to the health of our microbiome. The

GMO story starts with Roundup, an herbicide developed in 1974 by Monsanto, a giant agriculture biotech company based in St. Louis, Missouri. Roundup, a powerful weed killer, contains glyphosate, a potent and toxic herbicide. In 2015, the World Health Organization declared glyphosate "probably carcinogenic to humans." The International Agency for Research on Cancer (IARC), based in Lyon, France, came to the same conclusion after conducting a review of numerous studies on the link between glyphosate and cancer.[10]

Here's where the Roundup story takes a twist. Back in the '80s and early '90s, Monsanto scientists were working on developing crops that would have a specific immunity or resistance to Roundup. Monsanto didn't want to sell less Roundup, but if the research-and-development scientists could develop crops that were resistant to Roundup, then their herbicide could be more freely used in the fields because the cash crops would be left alone.

And that's how these first GMO crops came to be. By taking genes from one organism—usually a mutated virus—and inserting them into the DNA of the crops, Monsanto scientists produced crops that were higher, larger, denser, and more resistant to Roundup.

In 1996, Monsanto introduced its first Roundup Ready crop—soybeans—followed by corn in 1998. After that, you could say that these Roundup Ready/GMO crops spread like wildfire. In just twenty years, 94 percent of soybeans and 89 percent of corn grown on U.S. farmlands came from Roundup Ready/GMO crops. Since the late '90s, more crops have been genetically modified—cotton, sugar beets, and canola—and have been widely adopted. Now new "superweeds" are filling farm fields, leading to lower crop yields and even more toxic herbicides used to combat the Roundup-resistant weeds. In 2013, researchers from MIT published a study in the journal *Interdisciplinary Toxicology* declaring glyphosate the "most important causal factor in the celiac disease epidemic," citing more than 270 studies examining how the pesticide could be linked to the fourfold increase in celiac disease (as well as numerous other autoimmune conditions) over the past few decades.[11]

And, yet, Roundup remains.

Four-fifths of the foods that most Americans eat are likely from GMO crops, fruits, and vegetables grown in nutrient-depleted soils doused with pesticides. Seeing that rates of leaky gut are sky-high from one end of the country to another, what should you do?

I offer two action steps:

1. Go organic and go local.
2. Eat fermented and sprouted foods.

Going organic means saying good-bye to processed foods filled with additives, fillers, and ingredients with long, tongue-twisting names that belong in a scientific textbook. Going organic also means you begin replacing conventionally grown fruits, vegetables, and meat, and conventional dairy, with:

▶ organically grown fruits, vegetables, and grains that haven't been sprayed with chemical pesticides and herbicides
▶ dairy products and meats from grass-fed livestock that haven't received antibiotics and growth hormones
▶ prepackaged foods produced with organic ingredients, like flaxseed crackers or sprouted ancient grain bread

It's certainly easier to shop for organic foods than ever before. Farmer's markets are always my first choice, but you can certainly do quite well shopping at natural foods grocers like Whole Foods, Sprouts, and Trader Joe's. Even traditional grocers like Kroger, Publix, and Safeway are selling organic produce, and the world's largest retailer, Walmart, now stocks organic dairy and produce, as well.

But what about cost? As my friend Jordan Rubin likes to say, "You can pay the farmer now or the pharmacy later." Yes, organic food costs more—about 25 percent more—but I can't think of a better investment for good health.

If organic foods' superior taste isn't enough to get you to change your shopping habits, then consider how much better—in terms of nutrient value—organic foods are for the body. In a study published in the *Journal of Applied Nutrition*, organically and conventionally grown apples, pears, potatoes, wheat, and sweet corn were compared and analyzed for their mineral content over a two-year period.[12] The organically grown foods were:

- ▸ 63 percent higher in calcium
- ▸ 73 percent higher in iron
- ▸ 118 percent higher in magnesium
- ▸ 178 percent higher in molybdenum
- ▸ 91 percent higher in phosphorus
- ▸ 125 percent higher in potassium
- ▸ 60 percent higher in zinc

Shopping for and consuming organic foods provides one of the surest paths away from developing leaky gut. After making the switch to organic, it's time to think about the power of fermented foods.

— Fermented Foods —

Until the first refrigerators made their debut a century or so ago, no one had the option of storing their produce for weeks at a time. Foods didn't have a long shelf life because there was no shelf life. You ate fruits and vegetables when they were in season. To survive the rest of the year, you preserved fruits, veggies, and dairy products. One of the most effective, enduring, and beneficial of these preservation processes was known as fermentation.

In her book *Gut and Psychology Syndrome*, Dr. Natasha Campbell describes fermentation's long history:

"Every traditional culture, when you look at their traditional diet, fermented their foods. They fermented everything—dairy, grains, beans, vegetables, fruits, meats, and fish. When the cabbages were ripe in September, they made fermented cabbage. Perhaps for a month or two, they ate fresh cabbage, but then for the rest of the year, ten months of the year, they ate cabbage in a fermented form. Quite a large percent of all the foods that people consumed on a daily basis were fermented. And with every mouthful of fermented foods, they consumed trillions of beneficial bacteria."

The process of fermentation is actually very simple. Take this example of how cabbage is turned into a probiotic powerhouse: sauerkraut. Sauerkraut is made by a process called facto-fermentation. Beneficial bacteria live on the surface of all living plants, fruits, and vegetables.

Lactobacillus lives on the surface of cabbage. (You may recognize the name as it's also commonly found in yogurt.)

In order to make sauerkraut, you simply put shredded cabbage, water, and salt in a glass mason jar with the lid slightly turned so a small amount of air can escape for three to ten days at room temperature. The lactobacillus bacteria feed off the natural sugar found inside the cabbage and turn it into lactic acid, which acts as a natural preservative and is what gives fermented foods like yogurt, kefir, and sauerkraut their sour taste. Pretty simple, right? Cabbage, water, sea salt, and a glass jar is all you need.

Not only does the fermentation process allow the cabbage to keep for long periods of time, but it also results in higher levels of vitamins C and B than the original cabbage, as well as greater numbers of live lactobacilli and other beneficial microbes.

During the fermentation process, bacteria and yeasts break down proteins into amino acids, fats into fatty acids, and complex sugars into simple sugars such as glucose. Additional beneficial compounds are created during this process, including other probiotics that help feed the gut lining and maintain a healthy bacterial balance.

This fermentation process does more than preserve food—it also makes foods more absorbable by the body. In the case of sauerkraut, the amount of vitamin C becomes *twenty times* higher than in the same helping of fresh cabbage. This process turns not only cabbage into sauerkraut, but grape juice into wine, grains and water into beer, various vegetables into relish, and cow, goat, and sheep's milk into a variety of fermented dairy foods such as kefir, yogurt, and cheese.

Let's look at some of the most beloved fermented foods, which are some of the richest sources of beneficial bacteria.

For centuries, **kefir** (pronounced *KEE-fer*) has been prescribed in European and Asian folk medicine. Kefir is a fermented beverage made from the milk of cows, goats, or sheep, and is one of the foods I consume most often. I usually buy a plain goat's milk version at my local farmer's market every week and drink it with a bit of prebiotic-rich raw honey and sprouted flax meal. Even though I recommend goat's milk kefir to my patients, kefir from cow's milk is acceptable. Sheep's milk kefir is excellent, but even more difficult to find. If you have issues with dairy, try coconut kefir instead.

There's no doubt that kefir is one of the most microbe-rich foods in the world, with high microbial diversity of ten to thirty-four different strains of bacteria in each serving. Similar to yogurt but with a more liquid consistency, kefir is usually sold in ready-to-drink quart bottles at farmer's markets and natural foods stores. The tart-tasting, effervescent beverage contains high levels of naturally occurring bacteria and yeast, which break down the lactose in milk (making it suitable for those who are lactose intolerant). One of the many reasons many people today are lactose intolerant is that the modern practice of pasteurization kills off the beneficial bacteria and enzymes, but a study in the *Journal of the American Dietetic Association* showed that kefir improves lactose digestion and tolerance in adults with lactose malabsorption.[13]

Kefir is a great base ingredient to build smoothies around: just add eight ounces of kefir into a blender, an assortment of frozen berries or fruits, a bit of raw honey, and sprouted flax meal, and blend for a delicious, satisfying smoothie.

(Note: Exercise caution when purchasing commercial brands of kefir, which are often made from cow's milk, tend to be overly sweetened, and can contain excessive additives. Be sure to check the ingredients list.)

Research on **yogurt** has long underscored how helpful it is with supporting positive changes in the microflora of the gut and boosting the immune system through the action of two of the most common major genii of probiotics—lactobacillus and bifidobacterium. Most yogurt has one to three total strains of beneficial bacteria, about a tenth or a quarter of the number in kefir. While I prefer kefir, yogurt is still worthy of being included in any lineup of top probiotic foods. Because of its universal popularity, yogurt is a robust $7 billion industry in the United States. Just in the last year, more than six hundred new yogurt products came out on the market.

With so much market share at stake, major yogurt companies cut a few corners; most make their yogurt out of pasteurized milk from conventionally raised dairy cows fed with antibiotic-laced grains and corn. Shop for yogurt that's produced from grass-fed animals, preferably goats, followed by sheep, then followed by cows. Old Chatham Sheepherding Company is an organic brand that I recommend.

Raw cheese made from grass-fed cow's, goat's, and sheep's milk are particularly high in probiotics, including thermophillus, bifidus, bulgaricus, and acidophilus.

Raw cheese means that the cheese was made from milk that hasn't been pasteurized. When heated to 161 degrees Fahrenheit for thirty-one seconds (the process of pasteurization), the milk is sterilized, destroying not only many of the probiotics but also digestive enzymes. Pasteurization makes milk much more difficult for your body to digest and can contribute to inflammatory bowel disease, which is why I don't recommend pasteurized dairy products.

Raw milk isn't easy to find, even in states where it's legal. Thirty states allow raw milk to be sold with a variety of restrictions. However, you can buy raw cheese in every state of the union because the cheeses are aged for sixty days or longer. Raw cheese is readily available in natural grocers and health food stores everywhere.

Coconut kefir is a fermented version of coconut water and kefir grains. A nice stand-in for dairy, coconut kefir contains some of the same probiotic strains you'd find in traditional dairy kefir, but in lesser quantities. Coconut kefir is readily available in natural foods stores as well—but not on any shelves, as it must be refrigerated. Coconut kefir has a great flavor, especially with a bit of stevia, water, and lime juice.

Sauerkraut has a long history—chopped cabbage has been salted and fermented in its own juice for thousands of years, reputedly for Chinese laborers building the Great Wall of China. Today, sauerkraut is widely thought to be German in origin since *sauerkraut* is German for "sour cabbage." A staple in ethnic German restaurants in this country, sauerkraut gets a lot of upturned noses because of its bitter taste. That's too bad, because this fermented cabbage is high in organic acids, vitamin C, and digestive enzymes and is a superior source of natural lactic acid bacteria like lactobacillus. I tend to buy some cabbage or cucumbers at the market and then make my own sauerkraut or fermented veggies at home. (Don't forget the basic sauerkraut recipe I shared on page 118.)

Normally, I'd recommend pickles as a top probiotic food—but most brands of store-bought pickles (as well as commercial sauerkraut) should be avoided, as both foods are not naturally fermented. Instead, they're soaked in salt and vinegar to mimic the flavor of traditional sauerkraut and pickles. This processing technique is faster and cheaper, but results in the loss of many much-needed probiotics.

Kimchi is a kissing cousin to sauerkraut that's been gaining popularity in recent years. Originally from South Korea, kimchi is created by mixing Chinese cabbage with a mélange of foods and spices such as carrots, garlic, ginger, onion, sea salt, red pepper flakes, chili peppers, and fish sauce. The mixture is then set aside to ferment for anywhere from three days to two weeks.

Kimchi is seriously *spicy* but that hasn't stopped this condiment from becoming South Korea's national dish. Koreans serve kimchi at almost every meal, crediting this zesty pickled cabbage with fighting off the entire culture's infections and respiratory illnesses (a happy bonus of its being sky-high in vitamins A, B, and C as well as boasting all that lactobacillus). Research has found that kimchi lowers risks of heart disease, diabetes, and metabolic syndrome as well. A 2013 study in the *Journal of Medicinal Food* showed that participants who ate kimchi daily saw significant decreases in total glucose, total cholesterol, and LDL cholesterol (or "bad" cholesterol) after just one week of eating kimchi daily.[14]

After kefir, kimchi is my second-favorite probiotic food. I love its spicy mixture of cabbage, carrots, and radish. I typically add a dollop of kimchi over a serving of grass-fed barbecue beef, or I mix it into my stir-fry. Kimchi is also a great condiment with wild-caught salmon.

Natto is eaten over white rice for dinner *or* breakfast in Japan. Natto is made from fermented soybeans that contain the extremely powerful probiotic *Bacillus subtilis*, which has been shown in various studies to bolster the immune system, support cardiovascular health, and enhance digestion of vitamin K_2. Vitamin K_2 improves bone density by moving calcium around the body to where it's needed most, especially the bones and teeth. The *Bacillus subtilis* in natto may also improve immune function, according to an animal study published in the *Journal of Dairy Science*.[15]

You usually have to shop at Asian markets or well-stocked natural food stores to find this Japanese import. Those on a vegan diet should strongly consider adding natto, since this probiotic-rich food contains vitamin B_{12} and is one of the highest plant-based sources of protein for those who don't eat meat and dairy products.

Careful, though: natto is an acquired taste. The fermented soybean paste has an unappetizing smell reminiscent of Limburger cheese.

Miso may be familiar to you as the focus of soup served in Japanese restaurants in this country. Made from fermented soybeans, rice, or barley, miso soup is more palatable than natto but is more likely to be eaten at breakfast time in Japan because it's believed to stimulate the digestive system and energize the body for the day ahead. The fermentation process produces a rich, complex flavor of umami, also known as the "fifth taste" (the others being sweet, sour, salty, and bitter).

Kombucha has many people curious. The murky-looking trendy beverage with an exotic name is a combination of black or green tea, a dash of organic sugar or evaporated cane juice, and a fungus culture known as a "kombucha mushroom"—a pancake-shaped mass of bacteria and yeast that often appears as a mysterious blob floating in a bottle of kombucha.

Chinese in origin and tart as a Granny Smith apple, kombucha is loaded with a long list of beneficial bacteria, amino acids, B vitamins, and enzymes that deliver a cidery flavor with a kick of fizziness. If you've never tried kombucha, you're in for a bit of a surprise. The acidic tang takes a bit of getting used to, but don't let that stop you from giving this fermented beverage a try. Many claims have been made about kombucha, but its primary health benefits include digestive support, increased energy, and liver detoxification.

Kvass is a fermented beverage (pronounced *kuh-VAHSS*) has Eastern European roots that date from ancient times. Kvass hasn't caught on like kombucha but is steadily gaining popularity. Russian in origin, kvass has been traditionally made by fermenting rye or barley, which gives this cultured beverage a mild beer or ale flavor—minus the alcoholic content, however.

In recent years, kvass has been created with beets, an excellent food with an extensive nutritional profile. The fermentation process enhances the healthy benefits of beets and allows the nutrients to be readily absorbed by the body. You may have to shop online to find kvass made from beets or other root vegetables like carrots.

Finally, let me mention some other probiotic-rich favorites that count as probiotic foods, as long as you purchase the **organic fer-**

UNPASTEURIZED APPLE CIDER VINEGAR

We tend to think of prebiotics as something we crunch on—but how about something we drink? If it remains in its raw state, unpasteurized apple cider vinegar is a source of prebiotic pectin fiber. Apple cider vinegar also helps resistant starch convert into butyric acid, which supports healthy gut bacteria. Check for brands that still have "the mother"—a bloom of fermenting cellulose and acetic acid that boasts proteins, enzymes, and friendly bacteria—like my favorite brand, Bragg Apple Cider Vinegar.

---

mented versions: pickles, apple cider vinegar, ketchup, pickled ginger, and sourdough ancient grains, which are used for making bread. When fermented, these standards contain colonies of good bacteria that strengthen the immune system and cleanse impurities from the blood.

— Sprouting —

Another centuries-old process, sprouting not only makes grains and seeds easier to digest but makes their nutrients easier for the body to absorb as well. Sprouting deactivates a compound known as phytic acid, which is found on the coating of many seeds. Phytic acid can have a negative effect on the gut because it binds with minerals and blocks their absorption into the bloodstream. Phytic acid is an example of an *antinutrient* that naturally exists in grains, seeds, nuts, beans, and legumes. Other antinutrients include:

- ▶ **polyphenols,** which inhibit the healthy digestion of copper, iron, zinc, and vitamin B_1, along with enzymes, proteins, and starches found in plant foods.
- ▶ **enzyme inhibitors,** which prevent adequate digestion and upset the gastrointestinal tract. Enzyme inhibitors not only cause digestive problems, but they can also contribute to allergic reactions and mental illness.
- ▶ **lectins and saponins,** which irritate the gastrointestinal tract, leading to immune responses like joint pain and rashes.

Antinutrients have protective properties that help plants ward off pests and insects. When predators ingest antinutrients in plant materials, they don't feel so good. It stands to reason, then, that when humans eat grains, seeds, and nuts with antinutrients, our GI response interferes with our ability to digest the vitamins and minerals within the plants.

To neutralize the effects of antinutrients like phytic acid, we can ferment seeds and grains through sprouting, which involves soaking grains, nuts, seeds, legumes, and beans and then letting them dry so that they become easier to digest and our bodies can access their full nutritional profile. According to a medical study published in *Critical Reviews in Food Science and Nutrition*, when comparing the seeds in sprouted grains to unsprouted grain seeds, the unsprouted grains had "lower protein content, deficiency of certain essential amino acids, lower protein and starch availabilities, and the presence of certain antinutrients."

Sprouting grains also makes them easier to digest for people with gluten sensitivities. In a study published in the *Journal of Agriculture and Food Chemistry*, researchers sprouted wheat kernels for up to one week while analyzing them at different stages to observe the changes in gluten concentrations and nutrient levels.[16] They found that sprouting the wheat decreased the gluten proteins substantially, while increasing dietary fiber by 50 percent.

When choosing bread, look for the term "sprouted" on the label. I don't eat bread very often, but when I do, I like Ezekiel 4:9 Sprouted Grains bread, which is extremely high in fiber. Organic sourdough breads can be healthy and nutritious as well.

— Toxins in Our Homes —

In an effort to make our conventional food better suited to grocery stores and supply chains, the industrial agriculture (or "Big Ag") industry uses toxic pesticides to produce those perfect-looking but not very good-tasting tomatoes we talked about earlier. But in addition to those toxins, there are more than eighty thousand largely untested chemicals that have been introduced into our environment in the past fifty years, all in the name of progress and convenience—and all of which drives us a little further away from coexisting with dirt. We use plastic to cover our leftovers and stick them in the fridge. We buy Teflon pans so we don't have to scrub them. We make microwave popcorn so we don't have to heat all that oil and make a mess.

All of these thousands of chemicals combine in repeated toxic microexposures that accumulate daily on a cellular, systemic, even genetic level—including the bacteria in our guts. Remember my young patient Blake, from chapter 3? His diet played a major role in his inflammatory health condition, but it wasn't the only thing causing his skin issues and leaky gut—the industrial cleaners his mother used around the home were adding to his toxic load and weakening his gut even further.

Remember, it's not only what we eat but also what we touch. Everything we press, tap, rub, or nudge sheds microbes or other molecules that are quickly absorbed through our pores and directly into the bloodstream. Our body's largest organ, the skin, is the first line of defense for our immune system—which leaves it vulnerable to the chemical onslaught as well.

According to the Environmental Working Group (EWG), women use an average of twelve personal care products daily; men, six.[17] Your average grooming ritual might include soap, deodorant, toothpaste, shampoo, hair conditioner, lip balm, sunscreen, body lotion, shaving products (for men and women), and makeup (for women). And if you have children, you probably rub diaper cream, shampoo, lotion, and sunscreen on your hands before applying to their bodies. Just using these personal care products, women are exposed to a daily average of 168 chemical ingredients, and men to 85. But if you're cleaning in the kitchen and around the house, you're also exposing yourself to cleaning products like dishwasher detergent, laundry detergent, floor cleaner, furniture polish, glass cleaner. Each one of those negative microexposures is another opportunity for your microbiome—and your gut lining—to take a toxic hit.

A survey by the National Institute of Occupational Safety and Health analyzed 2,983 chemicals in personal care and cleaning products and determined that:[18]

▸ over 800 were toxic
▸ nearly 800 caused *acute* toxicity (triggering a rapid reaction)

- ▸ 314 caused a biological mutation in the living system of the body
- ▸ 376 caused skin and eye irritation
- ▸ 148 could cause tumors in laboratory animals
- ▸ 218 caused reproductive complications

Toxin overload is one of the main causes of leaky gut. When the gut gets inflamed over time, the tight junctions degrade and leave you more vulnerable to food particles, environmental chemicals, and bacterial waste leaking from your digestive tract and traveling into your body. While listing all of the most problematic household toxins could probably be a book in itself, here are a few of the most common:

- ▸ **Sodium laurel sulfate (SLS) and sodium laureth sulfate (SLES).** This duo can be found in 90 percent of all shampoos and many cosmetics, toothpastes, and hair conditioners. SLS and SLES are known as surfactants, meaning they reduce surface tension in products. These toxins can irritate the skin for up to a week, causing inflammation and damaging healthy skin oils. In a study published in *International Archives of Allergy and Immunology*, Canadian researchers found that exposure to surfactants significantly increases the permeability of the mucous layer and actively disbands and separates tight junctions.
- ▸ **Parabens.** Also commonly found in lotions, shampoo, shaving gels, makeup, and many other personal care products, parabens are readily absorbed into the body and affect hormonal balance, sparking scientific debate and studies regarding the risk of breast cancer and male reproductive problems.
- ▸ **Phthalates.** These chemicals lengthen the shelf life of cosmetics, hair spray, mousses, and fragrances. Phthalates damage the liver, kidney, and lungs, affecting the body's ability to process toxins. About one billion pounds of this chemical toxin are produced annually.
- ▸ **VOCs.** Volatile organic compounds are common petroleum-based chemicals that are neurotoxic and are present in perfumes, aftershave lotions, toiletries, shampoos, household cleaners, furniture polishes, and air fresheners.

▶ **DEA.** Diethanolamine (DEA), used as an emulsifier and foaming agent in shampoos, toothpaste, and bubble bath, is a hormone-disrupting chemical that has been linked to stomach and esophageal cancer in laboratory animals. It's telling that DEA has been banned in Europe but is still permissible in the United States.

▶ **Triclosan.** We've talked about this one before. The Environmental Protection Agency has labeled triclosan a pesticide, but we know it as the "active ingredient" in antibacterial soaps, body washes, and toothpaste. Triclosan is proven to accumulate in body tissues, leading to kidney and liver issues, yet it's been added to many consumer products to reduce or prevent bacterial contamination. Triclosan is also found in products ranging from kitchenware and furniture to clothing and toys. Way back in 2004, British researchers demonstrated that triclosan made *E. coli O157* antibiotic resistant after just two "sublethal" exposures—in other words, enough to hurt it, but not enough to kill it. Once it acquired that resistance, the *E. coli* was able to resist many other antimicrobial agents, including chloramphenicol, erythromycin, imipenem, tetracycline, and trimethoprim, as well as a number of biocides.[19] (Hmm, I wonder what's happened in the decade since?)

▶ **Chlorine.** Commonly used in municipal water systems as well as backyard pools, chlorine is also found in many household cleaners. A recent study published in the journal *Water Research* found that chlorinating water not only increased the prevalence of antibiotic resistance among known bacteria, it also increased the number of brand-new antibiotic-resistant genes. That's right: our drinking water is actively encouraging the evolution of antibiotic resistance.

This, as I mentioned before, is just a partial list. Consider that you likely run into these seven classes of chemicals daily—along with dozens more. Your goal should be to minimize your exposure to potentially harmful toxins that are proven to not only damage your gut lining and create antibiotic resistance, but affect your body's endocrine system, leaving your thyroid, pancreas, and adrenal glands even more vulnerable than before.

— Solve It with Essential Oils —

One of the ways I suggest my patients stay clean and use proper sanitation—yet not go overboard—is by choosing natural plant-based products such as **essential oils.** These aromatic compounds are extracted from plants that contain gentle antimicrobial properties. For example, tea tree oil, also known as melaleuca, has 327 medical studies to date proving its benefits as a gentle topical antimicrobial. A little tea tree oil mixed with water or coconut oil is a much safer hand sanitizer than the bottles of brightly colored gel you'll find at the drugstore.

Essential oils are extracted directly from the bark, flowers, fruit, leaves, seeds, or roots of a plant or tree. A steaming process distills the oil, separating it from water-based compounds. Even one drop of one of these highly concentrated oils can have a powerful health benefit. The reason I say *highly concentrated* is that it takes 150 pounds of lavender flowers to make only sixteen ounces of lavender essential oil and sixty-five pounds of red rose petals to make just a single fifteen-milliliter bottle of rose essential oil—which can sell for up to a thousand dollars! Think about those incredible ratios when you purchase a small vial of essential oil.

Essential oils have very small molecules that easily penetrate your cells. These molecules differ from fatty oils made from vegetables and nuts, which are much larger and cannot penetrate your cells, so they aren't therapeutic in the same manner. When you apply vegetable oils to the skin, they can clog your pores. Essential oils, on the other hand, are transdermal and will soak right into your skin.

Check out the Eat Dirt recipes on page 245 for step-by-step instructions on how to make everything from toothpaste to toilet cleaner using essential oils. Once you learn how easy and pleasurable—and inexpensive!—nontoxic home and body care products made with essential oils can be, you'll be hooked.

BONUS: For more DIY home remedies and recipes with essential oils you can download my eBook as a free bonus at: www.draxe.com/DIY-Guide

TEFLON: THE TIME SAVER THAT COULD BE KILLING US

Pots and pans coated with Teflon or nonstick surfaces are potential health hazards. The chemical that creates its trademark surface—perfluorooctanoic acid (PFOA)—releases toxins when heated. And what else do you do with cookware but heat it?

In fact, DuPont, the maker of Teflon, has commissioned its own studies that show that when Teflon is heated to 680 degrees Fahrenheit, six dangerous gases are released, two of which are known carcinogens. If 680 degrees sounds hot to you, it is, but the Environmental Working Group determined that a Teflon pan can reach 721 degrees Fahrenheit in just five minutes.

To protect you and your family, I recommend these safe cookware choices:

- ▶ stainless steel
- ▶ cast iron
- ▶ ceramic
- ▶ glass bakeware

These tried-and-true kitchen cookware choices have stood the test of time. Add a little butter or healthy coconut oil in the pan and start cooking. Sure, you'll have to pay more attention to foods sticking to the surface, but it's well worth it in the long run to protect your family from toxins.

— Gut Protectors: Practice Earth-Friendly "Chemistry" —

You can begin to protect yourself against environmental toxins with these strategies. You'll learn more about each of these approaches as we move through part 2.

- ▶ **Organic foods are the healthiest foods on the planet.** You'll never go wrong when you fuel your body with food that hasn't been grown with pesticides and herbicides or raised in stockyards with antibiotics and hormones.
- ▶ **Fermenting foods** is not only a way to preserve foods but

an excellent way for your body to receive much-needed probiotics in the gut. Fermented vegetables such as sauerkraut, pickled carrots, and kimchi supply the gut with useful microorganisms.

▶ **Experiment with soaking and sprouting.** When grains, nuts, seeds, legumes, and beans are soaked or allowed to germinate, they transform into abundant nutritional sources with vitamin C and vitamins B_2, B_5, and B_6.

▶ **Consider doing a "makeover" of your home** or living space with your personal and skin-care products and home-cleaning products. Clean out your under-the-sink cabinets and medicine cabinets and replace those toxic products with nontoxic brands recommended on the Environmental Working Group website or stocked at your natural food store.

Living in a world with this much toxicity can certainly be stressful. Unfortunately, stress—all by itself—is a contributing factor of leaky gut. Let's look at how the nervous system in your gut factors into your health—and how taking care of yourself and slowing down might be the best thing you can do to repair your gut.

8

Our Stressful Lives

One of the biggest (and most often overlooked) causes of leaky gut is emotional and mental stress. Stress makes us sick, wears us out emotionally, and can exacerbate just about any health condition you can think of. In fact, more than 75 percent of all physician visits are for stress-related ailments—many of them related to the gut.

This is no coincidence. The mind-body connection is not a philosophy; it is a biological fact. The microbes and nerve cells in the gut communicate with each other and the brain constantly via what's known as the gut-brain-microbiota axis.[1] At the center of this axis is the vagus nerve, a thick bundle of nerves that runs along the spinal column, connecting the hundred million neurons in the gut's enteric nervous system to the base of the brain at the medulla.[2] This connection is at the root of that "butterflies in the stomach" feeling we get when we're excited—or the "kick to the gut" we feel when we're stressed.

In addition to this direct gut-brain connection, our millions of enteric nerves—collectively known as our so-called second brain—have their own receptors that react to the presence of certain gut bacteria and metabolites such as short-chain fatty acids. This second brain is responsible for producing 90 percent of the body's serotonin (the neurotransmitter of contentment that's known to soothe anxiety and depression), as well as more than 50 percent of our dopamine (the neurotransmitter associated with excitement, learning, and reward). When the microbial balance is off in our gut, pathogenic microbes can interfere with the production of these neurotransmitters in many ways, including gobbling up needed nutrients that support mood, and secreting toxic chemicals that interfere with hormone and vitamin synthesis. When we're not able to produce optimal levels of these neurotransmitters, we are more likely to experience heightened stress and a lifelong tendency toward mental health challenges such as chronic anger, addiction, anxiety, depression, and more.

These mechanisms operate in a constant feedback loop—the fewer good microbes you have, the fewer positive neurotransmitters, and the more pronounced your response to stress becomes. The more stress hormones you produce, the greater your inflammation, which further irritates your stomach lining, increasing your likelihood of developing leaky gut—which leads to increased levels of pathogenic bacteria and yeast overgrowth. A 2014 study published in the journal *Gut* found that emotional or psychological stress greatly increased the risk of leaky gut and inflammatory bowel disease.[3] Even short bouts of stress can trigger or worsen leaky gut. In one study, researchers monitored participants' stress response to a stressful event (in this case, public speaking) by measuring their cortisol levels, and then assessed their gut health. They found that the people who released the most cortisol in reaction to the stress also experienced the greatest change in their intestinal permeability.[4]

I believe one of the primary contributing factors to my mother's cancer diagnosis as well as her leaky gut was her propensity for chronic stress. She was the mother of three kids and worked five days a week teaching children with special needs. A devoted wife and mom, she drove us kids to after-school activities, cooked dinner most nights, and did the housekeeping.

Looking back, I don't know how she did it all. Because of her busy schedule and emotional stress, my mother constantly felt overwhelmed and struggled with exhaustion. It wasn't until the second time she was diagnosed with cancer that she followed my advice to not only change her diet but also make real changes to her life that would help reduce her stress. Besides devoting more time to her two favorite outdoor (and "dirt"-centric) hobbies—horseback riding and gardening—Mom also:

- Cut back on work hours until she eventually shifted to a part-time position with twenty hours a week
- Took Sundays off
- Exercised daily for thirty minutes
- Received massage therapy
- Took long walks in nature
- Watched funny movies with my dad

Giving herself permission to decompress was a big mental hurdle for my mom. But once she committed to this self-care, to grounding herself in nature and spending time disconnected from the rush-rush-rush world, her entire health picture changed.

Slowing down can be hard. (Believe me, I know!) We all want to live productive lives, but if we're not careful, we can push ourselves past our breaking point very easily. The gut is actually one of the first places in the body to experience the damaging effects of stress—and once the gut lining has been breached, the resulting inflammation can worsen the next stress response. Let's take a closer look at how stress affects our gut health throughout our lives.

— Stopping the Stress Cascade —

While chronic stress is harmful to our health, each of us owes our life to the body's innate stress response. Our ancestors reacted to a threat by fighting it or fleeing from it, which is how they survived long enough to reproduce. Without stress, we'd have gone extinct along with the dinosaurs.

Reacting to a threat causes our HPA—hypothalamus-pituitary-adrenal—system to release stress hormones that help our body systems prepare for battle. The stress hormones adrenaline and cortisol flood the body. Blood pressure, breathing, and heart rate increase; glucose is released into the bloodstream for ready energy. All digestive and immune system functions are suppressed or put on hold, to help your body focus on the situation at hand.

Now, during a real crisis, your actions would make good use of these processes. You would fight or flee, burning through your adrenaline and cortisol via physical exertion, using that extra glucose for a burst of speed. Once the threat subsided, you would experience a release of dopamine—your brain's reward for having survived the challenge. Thereafter, basking in the afterglow, you might take comfort by resting or spending time with loved ones. All of these actions would help to restore your metabolic and hormonal balances.

For many of us today, "fight or flight" is not an emergency survival mechanism but our default operating mode. Perhaps we think we perform better under pressure or thrive on deadlines, so we become literal adrenaline junkies, addicted to the motivating zoom of norepinephrine and the resulting release of dopamine. Soon our bodies adapt to invoke the same physiological response that our predecessors once needed to literally fight (or flee) for their lives for smaller and less dangerous triggers. Stress hormones flood our bodies when we're sitting in traffic, waiting in a long line, stuck in a meeting, or running late to pick up the kids from school.

The net result is that our bodies are constantly prepared for battle— and yet we rarely dispel those stress hormones or take restorative actions to calm ourselves down and regain our balance. We don't soothe ourselves or take the time to rest after a stressful event. Instead, we move on to the next stressful activity, and our bodies get the message that we're in a constant, low-grade state of emergency.

This pattern doesn't just spring up from bad habits or a lack of positive coping skills—in some of us, it is hardwired from birth or infanthood. Early life trauma can prime our systems to release more cortisol in response to stress, and animal studies suggest this can establish a pattern of intestinal permeability (and even migration of pathogenic bacteria into the liver and spleen) from an early age. In others, even subtle shifts in the microbiome at an early age could interrupt our body's normal development of a healthy HPA axis or brain-body connection. When this system isn't allowed to mature completely, it could alter the responsiveness of our brain-to-endocrine-system and brain-to-immune-system pathways for life. Whereas someone who had less familial stress and/or a more balanced microbiome early on would learn to roll with stress a little easier, those whose early home life was tumultuous, or whose baby guts were overpopulated with more anx-

ADAPT TO STRESS WITH ASHWAGANDHA

Ashwagandha is an adaptogenic herb popular in Ayurvedic medicine that has shown incredible results for lowering cortisol and balancing thyroid hormones, of particular concern to people with stress-related leaky gut. In India, ashwagandha is known as the "strength of the stallion" since it has traditionally been used to strengthen the immune system after illness.

More than two hundred studies[5] have investigated ashwagandha's effects and found it to:

▶ Reduce anxiety and depression
▶ Combat the effects of stress
▶ Increase stamina and endurance
▶ Prevent and treat cancer
▶ Reduce brain cell degeneration
▶ Stabilize blood sugar
▶ Lower cholesterol
▶ Boost immunity

Perhaps most helpful for those with leaky gut issues is ashwagandha's therapeutic power with thyroid issues. Ashwagandha can help people with both hypo and hyper thyroid issues, supporting a sluggish thyroid for people diagnosed with Hashimoto's, and improving the health of those with an overactive thyroid or Graves' disease. For anyone who's struggling with stress, lack of energy, adrenal overload, or thyroid issues, I recommend supplementing with 500 mg one to two times daily. You might also consider experimenting with similar adaptogenic herbs, such as holy basil, ginseng, and rhodiola.

ious bacteria, grow up to release more cortisol and experience greater inflammation in response to stress throughout their lives.

But let's say we did have a placid childhood, with happy bugs in our guts—are we safe? Well, we're certainly less prone to chronic stress—but we could experience a shift in our nervous system response at any moment in our lives. In addition to all of these stress-induced chemical responses—which can affect gut permeability—our use of antibiotics or any other gut-damaging factor we've discussed can tilt the microbial balance in our guts toward a dysfunctional stress response. Don't forget—that vagus nerve is ever vigilant, allowing the brain to interact and communicate directly with our microbes constantly. As we saw with those people who feared delivering a speech, any mental stress, either short or long term, can alter the bacterial composition of the gut, favoring "nervous" strains of bugs.

That's why stressful life events—a death in the family, lost job, divorce, or other trauma—often serve as triggers for autoimmune conditions. Countless studies have shown that depression is linked to health conditions such as irritable bowel syndrome, chronic fatigue syndrome, fibromyalgia, chronic pain, addiction, insulin resistance, and obesity. The hormonal shifts triggered by that acute stress encourage the proliferation of pathogenic bad bacteria and decrease beneficial probiotics, leading to higher rates of leaky gut—allowing those nervous bugs to spread anywhere in the body.[6]

HOW PATHOGENIC BUGS CHANGE OUR BEHAVIOR

All microbes learn, grow, adapt—and these adaptations actually have a hand in controlling our behavior. One thing they have the biggest control over is our food cravings. Bacteria help themselves survive by influencing us to choose foods that feature the particular nutrients they grow best on, rather than just taking whatever comes along.[8] Some bacteria love fat; others love sugar. The bacteria are able to manipulate our feelings and cravings by changing neural signals along the vagus nerve. In this way, our gut bacteria literally *teach us* what to eat—they're able to alter our taste receptors, release toxins that make us feel bad, and reward us with chemicals that make us feel good—all in the service of their own survival and population growth.

These mechanisms loop back on themselves constantly. We've all seen how stressful periods can have a domino effect on healthy habits. When we're stressed out, we often crave junk foods and eat poorly. All of that junk food wreaks havoc on the gut wall and the microbiome. We may have trouble sleeping, which has a devastating effect on our immune system, resulting in increased inflammation. Inflammation can produce toxic metabolites that can have a direct effect on brain function, with the potential to make any of us feel more jittery, anxious, and antisocial. The overabundance of cortisol in our bloodstreams greatly reduces the release of hydrochloric acid and the activity of digestive enzymes, effectively blocking your gut's ability to absorb nutrients.[7] The nerve cells in the gut that usually produce up to 95 percent of the body's serotonin are deprived of nourishment, so they don't have the tools to synthesize the very neurotransmitters that might help us feel better. Good bacteria starve and pathogens surge; our digestion suffers, we feel terrible, and we become even more stressed out.

Each version of this stress–inflammation–leaky gut cycle, no matter where it begins, can repeat itself endlessly and become self-perpetuating, unless we learn how to stop it. Thankfully, many of these same mechanisms can be reversed—we simply have to choose a place to break the cycle. Remember, the gut-brain communication channel works both ways: the gut talks to the brain, and the brain talks to the gut. We can address this from either end of that channel.

When we reduce stress, the composition of our microbiome becomes more balanced, which helps to repair the gut lining, which reduces inflammation, which reduces stress and anxiety. As the bal-

---

PROBIOTICS ALSO HELP WEIGHT LOSS

In addition to the numerous other benefits of probiotics, several have been proven to help promote weight loss. One of the most promising is *Lactobacillus rhamnosus*. An exciting study published in the *British Journal of Nutrition* found that, compared with women in the control group, overweight women who supplemented with *Lactobacillus rhamnosus* during a weight loss program showed significant reductions in fat mass and pathogenic bacteria. The researchers found the women continued to lose weight and fat mass even after the weight loss portion of the study had concluded, whereas those who'd not received the probiotics began to regain weight.[9] When seeking out a probiotic supplement, try to find one with a high colony count and several strains of bacteria—and if you're trying to lose weight, *Lactobacillus rhamnosus* certainly can't hurt.

ance of good bacteria increases, your mood and attitude will improve, leading you toward healthier habits and more gut-friendly foods. This positive feedback loop then gains momentum and continues to reinforce itself.

— Reinforcing the Good Guys —

One place to break the cycle is by reinforcing your good bugs. Research has proven that increasing good bacteria such as *Bifidobacterium longum*, through eating fermented foods or taking probiotic supplements, can actually reduce anxiety and stress.[10] *B. infantis 35624* has been shown to raise blood levels of tryptophan, the precursor to serotonin. Lactic acid–producing bacteria in yogurt also produce GABA, which activates the same neuroreceptors that are targeted by antianxiety drugs such as Valium and other benzodiazepines. One fascinating study published in the *Proceedings of the National Academy of Sciences* found that mice that had eaten the same amount of *Lactobacillus rhamnosus* as would be present in an average cup of yogurt lowered their cortisol levels by half. Faced with an anxiety-provoking test after ingesting the probiotic, the mice acted more daring and less nervous, behavior equivalent to what the researchers had previously seen when the mice were given antidepressant drugs.[11]

Since that study was published in 2011, researchers have found the same results in people, soothing everyone from babies with colic[12] to people who faced stressful work tasks[13] to people facing serious autoimmune conditions by altering their microbiomes with probiotics. A 2015 *Psychopharmacology* study found that even *pre*biotics—foods and supplements that feed beneficial bacteria in the gut—could have a similar effect on stress management. Women who were given a prebiotic supplement every morning for three weeks ended the experiment with lower cortisol levels than when they started.[14] In behavioral tests, they were also found to be less on edge, and when given a series of words they focused more on the positive words and paid less attention to the negative words. The effect could not be clearer: nourishing their guts nourished their minds.

Another way to interrupt the feedback loop is by combating stress at the source, by consciously and deliberately soothing our frayed nerves. The vagus nerve—that nerve that facilitates brain-gut chatter—is also a direct line into our parasympathetic nervous system, a.k.a. the "rest and digest" system. The PNS is responsible for helping the body recover from the fight-or-flight response—it lowers cortisol levels, reduces blood pressure, and directs blood back to the digestive tract. We humans are actually meant to spend much more time in PNS mode than we do. That's the mode that allows for peaceful contentment and joyful connection with our loved ones.

We can soothe our entire nervous system—literally teach our body to turn down our chronic stress response—when we choose activities that support the PNS, such as focused exercise, meditation, and prayer. By consciously tuning into that silent space within, we not only decrease our stress in the moment, we fortify our mind and our nervous system for the future. Research has found that toning the PNS can help turn down the inflammatory response in autoimmune conditions such as rheumatoid arthritis.[15]

Other relaxing activities can help tone the PNS, too. Taking long, deep breaths and making physical contact (like a big, long hug from a close friend) can trigger the vagus nerve and help to support the function of the PNS. (Even making that "blub, blub, blub" sound with a finger on the upper lip that we do with little babies has been shown to engage the PNS!)[16]

Any relaxing activity that helps flood you with a sense of safety, peace, and contentment can do the trick. Regular, ideally daily, engagement of your PNS, using any of these healing practices or others you might devise, will gradually teach your nervous system to bounce back more quickly from stress and increase your physical, emotional, and spiritual resilience. (See the list below for more ideas on how to soothe your stress response.)

I understand that stress is inevitable and often invites itself into our lives without warning. There have been times when I've felt that I'm passing through life arm in arm with stress. I've had to make adjustments. You can, too. Managing stress is all about taking charge of your lifestyle, your emotions, and the way you deal with problems. Until you take steps to move the needle of your stress level, symptoms of leaky gut are apt to hang around. But once you've begun your trip back from chronic stress, you'll find you're less inclined to use stress as a motivational tool, and more likely to seek out other, healthier ways to stay focused.

— Gut Protectors: Regular Stress Relief —

You'll learn more about stress relief in chapter 10, but please feel free to begin these or other stress relief measures *today*.

▸ **Take healing baths with lavender oil and Epsom salts.** A detoxifying bath is one of the best ways to relieve stress. Add twenty drops of lavender oil and one cup Epsom salts to a hot bath and soak for twenty pleasurable minutes. Then sip from a warm glass of chamomile tea. Drinking herbal teas of chamomile, nettle leaf, and dandelion will calm and relax you.

▸ **Exercise for at least thirty minutes every day.** Take your pick— Pilates, yoga, barre, weight training, Spin class, interval training, running, walking, or swimming—they're all great stress relievers. For extra motivation, make an exercise appointment with a family member, friend, or group of friends to exercise together at a certain time. The socialization part of exercise can be just as beneficial as the physical exertion.

▸ **Sit quietly for at least ten minutes a day.** Let your mind and body destress with meditation, prayer, or visualization. You may choose guided forms of any of these activities, or practice them on your own. Practicing gratitude by taking stock of all of the good things in your life—everything for which you feel grateful—can also yield profound health benefits.

▸ **Take a break from work and carve out time to socialize.** Just as you're expected to show up for work at certain times, you also need to schedule "fun times" or "relaxation times" during the week. Lots of type-A go-getters don't get enough rest, which is toxic to the liver. Be sure to arrange a complete day of rest each week, like on a Saturday or a Sunday.

▶ **Take a walk in nature and breathe deeply.** Walk for at least thirty minutes outside while deliberately taking deep, cleansing breaths of fresh air. Practice deep breathing by inhaling through your nose for five seconds, holding for three seconds, and then exhaling over five seconds through your mouth.

▶ **Don't try to do too much.** I urge you to do anything you can to slow down. That doesn't necessarily mean you have to sit on a park bench and watch the world go by, but cutting back on "life" in the short term can pay big dividends down the road. Give yourself time to rest and recharge, and your mind (and your gut) will thank you.

▶ **Consider some extra nutritional support.** When you've been pushing yourself to the limit for a while, your body is likely coming up short on several key nutrients necessary to help you cope. Consider adding vitamin D, vitamin B_{12}, and omega-3 fatty acid supplements to your daily regimen. Our body requires more of each of these nutrients during times of chronic strain, so supplementing each can play a critical role in improving symptoms of depression, stress, and anxiety. (And don't forget to get your vitamin D and some dirt simultaneously with extra time outdoors.)

Lowering your stress levels will make everything easier—as your "happy" gut bacteria and parasympathetic nervous system rebound, you'll likely find it much easier to adopt new self-care habits that will make you feel even better. I hope that you'll spend some of that time outdoors, to reclaim the lost connection that holds so much promise for our health. In the next chapter, we'll look at how modern-day medications have taken us far away from traditional remedies that were often more effective—and certainly friendlier to our gut microbiome.

9

Medication Nation

June and her son Ben came to see me when Ben was six years old. He'd been diagnosed with a learning disorder and autism. June told me that Ben had been developing normally until he was about two years old, when he got an ear infection.

For the next year, he was on mega doses of antibiotics, one after the other—but nothing would control his infections.

By the time he was six, Ben was only saying three words, total: "yes," "no," and "Mom."

As we watched Ben line up his toy cars on my examining table, we talked through some suggested changes. June left with her marching orders, and when they came back in two weeks, she was elated.

"After just a few days on the program, I walked into his bedroom one afternoon, and he turned around and said the first full sentence of his entire life," she said. "He's talking, really talking—he's gone from two words to forty words in the past two weeks."

Working with Ben was an ongoing process. Because of his sensory issues, he was extremely restricted in what he ate. When he first came to me, he was only eating one food—chicken nuggets. And only one specific brand.

The first thing we did was shift to a gluten-free/dairy-free diet. That took a little bit of adjusting because of Ben's restricted eating. But June stuck with it and together we devised a homemade chicken nugget using organic chicken and almond flour for the "breading." He would also eat french fries, so we gradually switched him over to sweet potato fries, cooked in coconut oil and sea salt. Ben also began to drink smoothies, which was a blessing because we could squeeze some different foods in there without his really knowing. We made those smoothies with fruit, collagen powder, probiotic powder, and coconut milk. Occasionally, he would acquiesce to eat chicken bone broth soup with carrots.

Although this was not a very diverse diet, Ben was getting so much more nutrition than before that we considered it a huge win. Even more important than what he was eating was what he *wasn't* eating—the gluten and dairy that had been harming his gut.

As soon as he could tolerate swallowing pills, we started him on a regimen of probiotic capsules, digestive enzymes, fish oil, and a B-complex vitamin. June was committed to the Eat Dirt philosophy. She swapped out all their household cleaners with essential-oil-based cleansers. She had a diffuser for essential oils in the house, and together we created blends to help support a more serene environment for Ben. We also created an essential oil blend from frankincense, vetiver, chamomile, and cedarwood that June dabbed onto Ben's neck before school to help him stay calm and focused.

I continued to see Ben for about five years. I ran into June in the grocery store recently, and she told me that he was doing great. His diagnosis had changed from moderate to severe autism to high-functioning autism/Asperger's subtype. He'd transferred from his adaptive school back to their neighborhood school, and he was able to transition into a full-inclusion classroom. "If you met him today, you might think he was just a bit quirky," June said.

But I will never forget how, in the midst of our treatments, June had broken down and confessed to me how frustrated she had been with the pediatrician and ear, nose, and throat specialist who'd treated Ben during that year of his ear infections. "How could they not know?" she asked tearfully. "I told them I was concerned, I told them about how much he was changing. How could they keep giving him all those antibiotics and not think there'd be any repercussions?"

— The Collateral Damage of the War on Bugs —

We've come to the last of the five gut grenades, and possibly the worst.

This may come as a surprise to you, but the number-one cause of leaky gut is our modern medical system. Prescription medications—the biggest weapon in modern medicine's arsenal—readily deplete the body of nutrients and damage the gut lining. This is why *all* synthetic drugs in some way cause leaky gut.

People don't realize how some of the most popular drugs in America rob the body of essential vitamins, minerals, antioxidants, and probiotics . . . which leads to common symptoms such as fatigue, depression, and pain . . . which leads to more serious diseases and additional rounds of prescription drugs.

Perhaps the most dramatic example of this downward health spiral is our country's epidemic of addiction to prescription pain medication. Often people reach for these drugs as a relief from chronic pain caused by autoimmune conditions such as fibromyalgia, lupus, or MS. These medications act on the opioid receptors in several places within the body, including the gut, which interferes with peristalsis and blocks the release of digestive enzymes, really complicating digestion.[1] People on opioids tend to suffer from GERD and acid reflux, as well as debilitating constipation, which then leads to long-term laxative use.[2]

What makes all of this even sadder is the fact that these incredibly dangerous drugs just aren't that effective long term. A Danish study of more than eleven thousand patients found that long-term opioid users were more likely to have lower quality of life, be unemployed, be in poor health, have spent more time and money on health care—and still were more likely to describe themselves as experiencing moderate to severe to very severe pain.[3]

Suzy Cohen, RPh (registered pharmacist) and author of *Drug Muggers*, believes that more than half of the prescribed drugs approved in the United States commonly deplete specific nutrients in the body. She likened this phenomenon to a "mugging" that many are not aware of, just like having their pockets picked in a crowded subway. According to Cohen, prescription drugs can mug you by:

- altering the acidity in your stomach
- overburdening your liver
- damaging your intestinal lining
- inhibiting enzymes involved in turning nutrients into more usable substances

Certain drugs require specific nutrients in order to work, which can lead to deficiencies. The medications that have proven to be the most problematic are NSAIDs (Advil, Aleve, Celebrex), proton pump inhibitors (Prilosec, Prevacid), thyroid medications, and—you guessed it—antibiotics.

Here's a look at some of the most common drugs and the vitamins, minerals, nutrients, and beneficial microbes they either diminish or completely deplete:

TYPE OF DRUG	EXAMPLES	NUTRIENTS DIMINISHED OR DEPLETED
Antacids	Pepcid, Prilosec, Tagamet, Zantac, Prevacid	Calcium, folic acid, iron, vitamin B_{12}, vitamin D, zinc
Antibiotics	Amoxicillin, penicillin, sulfonamide, erythromycin	*Bifidobacteria bifidum* and *Lactobacillus acidophilus* (friendly beneficial bacteria), vitamins B_1, B_2, B_3, B_6, B_{12}, vitamin K, calcium, magnesium, potassium
Antidepressants	Adapin, Aventyl, Evavil, Tofranil	Coenzyme Q10, vitamin B_2
Antidiabetic drugs	Dymelor, Micronase, Tolinase, Glucophage	Coenzyme Q10, vitamin B_{12}
Anti-inflammatory drugs	Aspirin, Advil, Aleve, Motrin, Naprosyn, Orudis, Voltaren	Folic acid, iron, potassium, vitamin C

(*continued on next page*)

TYPE OF DRUG	EXAMPLES	NUTRIENTS DIMINISHED OR DEPLETED
Anti-inflammatory drugs (stronger)	Cortisone, dexamethasone, hydrocortisone, prednisone	Calcium, folic acid, magnesium, potassium, selenium, vitamin C, vitamin D, zinc
Blood-pressure-lowering drugs	Bumex, Edecrin, Lasix	Calcium, magnesium, potassium, sodium, vitamin B_1, vitamin B_6, vitamin C, zinc
Cholesterol-lowering drugs	Baycol, Lescol, Lipitor, Mevacor, Zocor	Coenzyme Q10
Hormone replacement therapy	Premarin, Prempro	Magnesium, vitamin B_6, folic acid, vitamin C, zinc
Oral contraceptives	Estrostep, Norinyl, OrthoNovum, Triphasil	Folic acid, magnesium, vitamin B_2, vitamin B_3, vitamin B_6, vitamin B_{12}, vitamin C, tyrosine, zinc
Thyroid replacement	Synthroid	Calcium
Tranquilizers	Ormazine, Mellaril, Prolixin, Thorazine, Haldol	Coenzyme Q10, vitamin B_2

Not only do prescription medicines drain the body of nutrients and contribute to leaky gut, they can make some of its other symptoms, such as inflammation, much worse. Note that we're not just talking about prescription medications here—even those over-the-counter drugs, like aspirin, ibuprofen, and antacid medications, that we sometimes take without a second thought cause damage to the mucosal lining of the small intestine. But one of the surest ways to prevent serious harm to the lining of the small intestine by NSAIDs is simply to stop using them.

The risk with prescription medicines goes way beyond leaky gut, unfortunately. In an editorial published in the *Journal of the American Medical Association*, Barbara Starfield, MD, of the Johns Hopkins School of Hygiene and Public Health, reported that 290 people a day—

approximately 106,000 a year—*die* from nonerror, adverse effects of medications. Dr. Starfield noted that figure was for deaths only and did not include adverse effects associated with disability or discomfort.[4]

Compare this number to the top two leading causes of death in this country. According to the Centers for Disease Control and Prevention, 611,105 people died from heart disease and 548,881 people succumbed to cancer in 2013.

All of this extremely troubling data just begs the question: what's the number of people who die each year from taking nutritional supplements, herbs, or essential oils?

Answer: a resounding *zero* in 2013, according to the annual report from the American Association of Poison Control Centers.[5] That is an incredible statistic when you consider that U.S. citizens alone took over sixty *billion* vitamin and mineral doses that year.

In fact, there haven't been any recorded deaths from consuming nutritional supplements in many years, according to the Centers for Disease Control and Prevention. That means no deaths from taking calcium, magnesium, chromium, zinc, selenium, iron, and silver, no fatalities from taking blue-green algae, medicinal mushrooms, melatonin, or any homeopathic remedy, and no deaths from taking herbal products like echinacea, oregano, ginseng, or ginkgo biloba.

Will people sometimes have a reaction to natural remedies? No doubt. Anything we ingest has the capacity to give us a reaction, whether it's a controlled narcotic or a capsule of bee pollen—or a whole wheat bagel! But rather than throw all our faith into big-gun pharmaceuticals, I think we need to broaden our interpretation of "medicine."

— Going to the Well Once Too Often —

Of all the ways we diminish our gut flora with medications, by far the most devastating practice is the overuse of prescription antibiotics. When you make an appointment with your family physician after catching the flu bug, getting hit with a nagging cough, or being bothered by a respiratory ailment, it's likely that you'll walk out of the examination room holding a prescription for amoxicillin or cephalexin. Antibiotic prescriptions are ubiquitous and rising fast worldwide. A 2014 survey funded by NIH, the Bill and Melinda Gates Foundation, and Princeton University looked at antibiotic prescriptions in seventy-one countries. They found that global consumption of antibiotics rose over 35 percent between 2000 and 2010.[6]

I was no different growing up. When frigid temperatures hit central Ohio every January, I couldn't shake a nagging cough, which seemed to necessitate a prescription for antibiotics. My mother relied on the traditional medical system to keep us healthy, as do millions of parents. Unfortunately, the CDC estimates that upwards of 50 percent of antibiotics prescribed for upper respiratory infections are prescribed incorrectly.[7] A 2015 study published in the journal *Gut* found that the three most common outcomes of antibiotic abuses are:

▸ Elimination of beneficial microbial species in the gut, including some that never return.
▸ Damage to tissues and organs of the body, especially the small intestine, large intestine, stomach, and liver.
▸ Antibiotic resistance, making future infections more difficult to treat.

While antibiotics are an important tool in fighting life-threatening bacterial infections, and they have saved patients from the ravages of everything from pneumonia to open flesh wounds, we now know that the indiscriminate and widespread use of antibiotics leaves our digestive tracts vulnerable to even *more* bugs while promoting the spread of antibiotic resistance. Bacteria can mutate in just days—or even hours. With the scale of that many bacteria, changing that quickly, it's no wonder some of our rudimentary, antiquated antibiotics are becoming ineffective against them. Once any one strain of pathogenic or neutral bacteria grows too populous, they achieve quorum sensing.

Quorum sensing is what brought us the scourge of antibiotic resistance. Together, strains of bacteria develop strategies to bolster their numbers and change their genetic code so they don't have to be victims of certain antibiotics any longer. In the last fifty years, bacteria have increasingly gained the power to shrug off antibiotics. Infections now exist that have become almost impossible to treat. One of the most devastating is *Clostridium difficile*, which has been rendered almost entirely antibiotic resistant. More than fifteen thousand people die of *C. diff* every year. Most cases are contracted after a course of broad-spectrum antibiotics, such as fluoroquinolones, cephalosporins, clindamycin, and penicillins, that wipe out a huge portion of your gut population—except *C. diff*.[8] Given this power vacuum, the *C. diff* population explodes and overtakes the gut, producing toxins that attack the intestinal lining.

Every year, American doctors write about a hundred million antibiotic prescriptions for conditions that drugs can't treat.[9] In part, that's because 36 percent of Americans incorrectly believe antibiotics can cure

A *WHAT* TRANSPLANT?

Perhaps the greatest irony of the antibiotic resistance crisis is the treatment that holds the most promise to cure it: the "fecal microbiota transplant," a.k.a. a poop transplant.

It may sound gross, but the procedure is actually very simple and very "clean." Fecal matter contains the highest concentrated source of gut bacteria—up to half of the mass of our waste is composed of bacteria. For a transplant to occur, a fecal donor is first screened for any diseases or infections, then makes a "donation." That specimen is introduced into the sick patient, either via a tube during a colonoscopy or by mouth, in a series of thirty enteric-coated capsules.

One dose of FMT has been shown to be 92 percent effective against recurrent *C. diff* within just a few days.[10] These were patients at death's door— yet they sprang out of bed, completely healed, practically overnight. Some scientific trials actually had to be stopped because the fecal transplant was shown to be so effective, the researchers decided it was not ethical to deny the control group that same lifesaving intervention.

More FDA trials are currently under way, and the medical community is hopeful about the lifesaving potential of this treatment. But already the pharmaceutical companies are racing to market with their own synthetic fecal matter—because of the supposed "ick" factor. They see, no doubt, the tremendous financial boon from this type of treatment. But haven't we learned? If nature provides us such an effective, safe solution, can't we just stop there—can't we get over the "ick" factor—to save our health?

viral infections like the common cold or flu.[11] By age two, the average child in the United States has taken about three courses of antibiotics. (Autistic children average twelve by age three.) That's essentially like dropping a hand grenade in a region of your body, knowing that you're going to kill some of the bad guys but also take out many of your own soldiers as well.

We should know better by now. We can do better. We need to start eating dirt, if not for our own health, then for the health of the entire world. One way we can do that is by consciously trying to replace some of our long-lost old friends with the beneficial microbes in probiotic supplements.

— Probiotics to the Rescue —

Probiotics are good medicine. Beneficial bacteria are not only responsible for protecting the gastrointestinal tract, they also support the liver in detoxification, the kidneys in cleansing, and the bowel in elimination. Beneficial microbes produce vital nutrients for the body like vitamins, minerals, and fatty acids as well as certain digestive enzymes that help the digestive system break down food. They affect important nerve cells that sense nutrients, measure acids, and trigger peristaltic waves that move digested food through the small intestine and into the large colon, where waste products are eventually expelled by the body. When our good bugs aren't properly fed or replenished, however, they eventually disappear and leave your immune system vulnerable to attack.

In many ways, probiotic supplements can either replace pharmaceutical and over-the-counter medications or help protect our inner ecosystem from medicine-induced collateral damage, especially in the areas of:

Digestive health. An analysis of eighty-two studies of probiotics' ability to alleviate diarrhea was conducted by RAND Corporation researchers in Southern California and published in the *Journal of the American Medical Association*.[12] Researchers found that probiotics reduced the risk of antibiotic-associated diarrhea by 42 percent. In a separate 2014 review by the Yale University School of Medicine, researchers found that probiotics shortened diarrhea attacks in children and reduced the incidence of diarrhea in adults.[13]

Vitamin B and vitamin B$_{12}$ levels. Probiotics increase levels of B vitamins, especially the all-important vitamin B$_{12}$, by improving nutrient absorption. A study published in the *Journal of Gastrointestinal Surgery* from the Stanford University School of Medicine showed that levels of vitamin B$_{12}$ were 50 percent higher in the patients taking a probiotic supplement compared to the control group after just three months.[14] (As I always say to my patients, *You aren't what you eat; you are what you absorb.*)

Respiratory infections. Nearly two hundred students living in dorms at Framingham State University in Massachusetts were given either a placebo or a powder blend containing probiotic strains during the height of the flu season. Researchers found that while all students caught colds or the flu bug at roughly the same rate, the students who took probiotic supplements experienced:[15]

▶ Colds that were two days shorter (four days versus six days)

▶ Symptoms that were 34 percent less severe

▶ Fewer missed days in the classroom (by half)

Mental health. Bacteria are able to manipulate our feelings and cravings by changing neural signals in the vagus nerve, a long column of a hundred million nerve cells that stretches from the gut to the brain. A study released by the Leiden Institute of Brain and Cognition at Leiden University in the Netherlands suggests that probiotics help to lift mood and can be a good way to fight anxiety or depression.[16, 17] The researchers said their results point to a use for probiotics as either a remedy or a preventative therapy for depression.

Weight loss. I've seen this happen time and again in my practice. Probiotics help make your intestinal walls less permeable, which means fewer molecules enter your bloodstream and lead to the inflammation that can cause or contribute to obesity and type 2 diabetes. In a study published in the *British Journal of Nutrition*, researchers from Laval University in Quebec showed that although they ate the same diet, women who took probiotic supplements lost 9.7 pounds on average, while women who took a placebo lost 5.7 pounds.[18] The study demonstrated that the intestinal flora of obese individuals differ from those of thinner people, which may be due to the fact that a diet high in fat and low in fiber promotes certain bacteria at the expense of others, according to the study's summary.

Cognitive function. UCLA researchers found that magnetic resonance imaging (MRI) scans of women who regularly consumed the beneficial bacteria in yogurt showed greater connectivity within the prefrontal cortex, the executive function area of the brain that helps us with planning, organizing, emotional control, and self-regulation.[19]

Women's health. A woman's vagina is a finely balanced ecosystem of good and bad bacteria, inhabited by a range of microbes from a pool of more than fifty species. The probiotic lactobacillus is the most common, particularly for healthy women. When the balance is off, however, the results are often an uncomfortable yeast infection or bacterial vaginosis (BV). A study published in *Interdisciplinary Perspectives on Infectious Diseases* showed that lactobacillus strains can disrupt BV and yeasts and inhibit the growth of urogential pathogens.[20]

And, of course, leaky gut! A study of male athletes published in the *Journal of the International Society of Sports Nutrition* found that the men who supplemented with probiotics saw significant improvements in leaky gut and had lower levels of protein oxidation, which decreases recovery time.[21]

To tap into these health benefits, and many others, it's essential to include more probiotic-rich foods in our diets. As a culture, we have gotten away from eating probiotic foods because they often have a tart, sometimes bitter taste. Instead, our taste buds have been trained to crave sweet and salty foods. It's time to embrace the power of sour and the benefits of bitter foods because these flavors are indicative of probiotics, organic acids, and other compounds that support the growth of microbes in the gut.

Wherever you are on your health journey, it's a great idea to ensure you're receiving appropriate nutritional support by taking supplements, which offer a concentrated source of nutrients that today's diet can't always provide. A good probiotics supplement can colonize the intestinal tract and crowd out disease-causing bacteria, viruses, and yeasts. A 2013 study in *Critical Reviews in Food Science and Nutrition* found that using probiotics both internally and externally may have great potential for preventing and treating skin diseases such as eczema, atopic dermatitis, acne, and allergic inflammation as well as in treating skin hypersensitivity and UV-induced skin damage and promoting wound protection.[22]

When it comes to choosing a superior probiotics nutritional supplement, it's important to note that there are different types of strains of probiotics. The benefits experienced with one microbial strain may be completely different from the health benefits seen from another. Certain strains of probiotics and microbes support immunity, others support digestion, and some even help burn fat and balance hormones.

While many companies are now producing probiotics, the majority of them are ineffective at best, for two reasons. One, they are produced from milk in an aerobic environment, and most of our gut bacteria are anaerobic. And two, most probiotic supplements today are destroyed by stomach acid before they ever get to your digestive tract.

The first thing you should do is read the product label, which should reveal the genus, species, and strain of the probiotic or microbe. The product should also give you the CFUs (colony-forming units) at the time of manufacturing. Be aware that the majority of probiotics can die under heat, so knowing the company has proper storage and cooling procedures is also important. You want to consider five specific things when buying a probiotic supplement:

- ▸ **Brand quality.** Look for brands that are certified organic.
- ▸ **High CFU count.** Purchase a probiotic brand that has a higher number of probiotics, ranging from fifteen billion to a hundred billion.
- ▸ **Strain diversity.** Search for a probiotic or microbiome supplement that has ten or more strains and contains not only probiotics but also SBOs, yeasts, fungi, and algae.
- ▸ **Survivability.** Look for strains like *Lactobacillus plantarum*, *Bacillus subtilis*, *Saccharomyces boulardii*, mushroom mycelia, phages, and other cultures or formulas that ensure that the probiotics make it to the gut and are able to colonize.
- ▸ **Research.** Do your homework and look for brands that have strains that support your specific needs. Check out these specific strains to see if any one meets your needs. (Most probiotic supplements are a blend of several strains.)

THE POWER OF PROBIOTICS

Here are just a few of the most commonly available probiotic strains and their proven therapeutic power.

Bifidobacterium bifidum—the most dominant probiotic in infants and in the large intestine. Supports production of vitamins in gut, inhibits harmful bacteria, supports immune system response, and prevents diarrhea.[23]

Bifidobacterium longum—supports liver function, reduces inflammation, removes lead and heavy metals.[24]

Bifidobacterium breve—helps colonize healthy gut community and crowd out bad bacteria.[25]

Bifidobacterium infantis—alleviates IBS symptoms, diarrhea, and constipation.[26]

Lactobacillus casei—supports immunity, inhibits *H. pylori*, and helps fight infections.[27]

Lactobacillus acidophilus—relieves gas and bloating, improves lactose intolerance. Shown to reduce *E. coli* by 61 percent, lower cholesterol levels,[28] and create vitamin K. Also important in GALT immune strength.

Lactobacillus bulgaricus—a powerful probiotic strain that has been shown to fight harmful bacteria that invade your digestive system and is stable enough to withstand the acidic digestive juices of the stomach. It also neutralizes toxins and naturally produces its own antibiotics.

Lactobacillus brevis—shown to survive the GI tract, boost cellular immunity, enhance natural T-killer cells, and kill *H. pylori* bacteria.[29]

Lactobacillus rhamnosus—supports bacterial balance and healthy skin. Helps fight urinary tract infections and respiratory infections, and reduce anxiety by reducing stress hormones and GABA neurotransmitter receptors.[30] Also survives GI tract.

Bacillus subtilis—an endospore probiotic that is heat resistant. Elicits a potent immune response and supports GALT.[31, 32] Suppresses growth of bad bacteria like salmonella and other pathogens.

Bacillus coagulans—an endospore probiotic that is heat resistant and improves nutrient absorption. Also has been shown to reduce inflammation and symptoms of arthritis.[33]

Saccharomyces boulardii—a yeast probiotic strain that restores natural flora in the large and small intestine and improves intestinal cell growth. It has proved effective in treating inflammatory bowel disease like Crohn's disease.[34] It's also been shown to have antitoxin effects,[35] be antimicrobial, and reduce inflammation.[36]

BONUS: If you want more advanced training on probiotics check out this bonus probiotic guide: www.draxe.com/probiotic-guide-bonus

Taking probiotic supplements can actually feel like you're taking medication, because the method of delivery—capsules—seems so similar. That confidence in "medicine" might be part of the reason why we have so much faith in them. But what about those remedies that are just as effective in the form that nature provided? A key aspect of what I hope to accomplish with *Eat Dirt* is to encourage us all to embrace the power of some natural remedies that actually have no corollary in Western medicine. Plants were our original medicines, after all, and nowhere is this link to ancient healing practices more real and tangible than with essential oils.

— Essential Oils for Healing —

We've talked about using essential oils in several different ways—as a home cleaner, in personal care products, even as a means of creating a serene environment. But as you learned in chapter 6, essential oils are some of humanity's oldest remedies, and remain among the most effective. Essential oils have antibacterial and antifungal benefits that are so well documented that the oils continue to be used in medical settings. Many oils massaged on the skin can heal or help treat skin conditions such as burns, cuts, or scrapes. Others may boost the immune system, help with insomnia, and aid with digestion.

All essential oils have unique compounds and healing properties, with many having multiple benefits and unique synergistic effects when used in combination. While I recommend that you work with a certified herbalist or doctor of naturopathic medicine to develop the right blends for you, I also want to share with you the scope of the power that's resting right there in the dirt! Here's a look at some of the most popular essential oils and how I use them with my patients.

Note: Essential oils are all about "good fit"—do you feel better when you smell them or wear them on your body? Don't force yourself to use a specific oil because you see your desired effect on this list. That's the beauty of essential oils—there are always, always other options, ones that will be more enjoyable for you. I promise! (See more material about essential oils on my website, DrAxe.com.)

Cedarwood was referenced by King Solomon as the fragrance that increases wisdom, and recent studies have proven this by demonstrating how cedarwood improves focus and memory.

Chamomile, a daisylike flower commonly used for herb infusions, has a calming effect on the body and helps with hormones and digestion. The gentle, comforting nature of chamomile benefits menstrual cramps, anxiety, and insomnia and can be used with children of all ages because of its soothing qualities.

Clary sage is the most beneficial oil for hormone balance and can be used for premenstrual syndrome relief. This essential oil also thickens hair and helps balance estrogen levels.

Clove, which comes from aromatic flowers native to Indonesia as well as India and Sri Lanka, provides antibacterial, antiparasitic, and antioxidant protection. Cinnamon oil has similar benefits and is exceptional for blood sugar balance.

Cypress improves circulation, reduces varicose veins, and can help heal broken bones.

Eucalyptus improves respiratory issues likes bronchitis, sinusitis, and allergies. This invigorating essential oil purifies the body and helps heal infections.

Frankincense builds immunity, reduces inflammation and age spots, increases spiritual awareness, and has powerful anticancer properties.

Geranium can help balance out both dry and oily skin, which makes it perfect for eczema, dermatitis, acne, and psoriasis. This oil, with its uplifting flowery scent, may decrease the appearance of wrinkles and can be used to reduce inflammation.

Ginger, known for its recognizable scent as well as its pungent taste, reduces inflammation, supports joints, improves digestion, and relieves nausea.

Grapefruit, a breakfast staple in some households, supports metabolism and cellulite reduction when mixed with coconut oil and applied topically to areas of cellulite.

Helichrysum, a flowering plant mainly found in South Africa, benefits cell regeneration, repairs damaged nerve tissues, and has anti-inflammatory qualities that heal swelling, bruises, and wounds.

Lavender helps with relaxation and sleep, lowers blood pressure, improves mood, and heals burns and cuts.

Lemon improves lymph drainage, cleanses the body, and works well in homemade cleaning products. Citrus oils such as orange and bergamot have similar benefits.

Lemongrass acts as a cleanser for the lymphatic system, functions as a natural deodorizer, and can also be used as a household cleaner. Lemongrass is also a natural bug repellent.

Myrrh, a natural antiseptic, can prevent or reduce infections. Myrrh also supports beautiful skin, reduces stretch marks, and improves hormone balance.

Oregano, a perennial herb, has powerful antimicrobial properties, helps kill fungi, and can help you kick a cold quickly.

Peppermint supports digestion, improves focus, boosts energy, reduces fevers and headaches, and offers muscle pain relief.

Rose is an extraordinary essential oil that reduces skin inflammation, lifts mood, and has an energizing scent.

Rosemary improves memory and naturally thickens hair, which makes this essential oil a welcome addition to homemade shampoo.

Sandalwood is a natural aphrodisiac that improves libido and can also improve energy. Sandalwood also has been shown to be effective against skin cancer and supports both male and female hormone balance.

Spikenard, an essential oil widely referenced throughout the Bible, can reduce stress, calm inflamed skin, stimulate the immune system, lower cortisol, and increase spiritual awareness.

Tea tree oil (melaleuca) is a natural antibacterial and antifungal essential oil that reduces bad odors and helps stimulate the immune system.

Thyme naturally improves levels of progesterone, which is needed by both women and men. This well-known essential oil is also beneficial for the immune system and respiratory system.

Vetiver, an Indian bunchgrass, helps calm the neurological system and has been proven effective in treating attention deficit disorder/attention deficit hyperactivity disorder, Parkinson's disease, dementia, brain injuries, and damaged nerve tissues.

Ylang-ylang—and that's not a typo—calms nerves and helps de-

AN EARTHY HEALING SCENT

Have you ever walked into a health spa room and been welcomed by the calming scent of orange blossoms or lavender?

If so, you experienced aromatherapy, a term coined by French chemist René-Maurice Gattefossé in 1928 after he used lavender oil to heal a burn on his hand. Intrigued at the success he enjoyed, Gattefossé investigated lavender oil's ability to treat other types of skin infections, wounds, and burns.

Aromatherapy has a variety of health benefits and is today viewed as an ideal noninvasive way to treat a variety of medical conditions. Traditional hospitals like Vanderbilt University Hospital use essential oils and aromatherapy in the treatment of anxiety, depression, and infections. A study published in *Perianesthesia Nursing* found that preoperative patients who received aromatherapy with lavandin oil were significantly less anxious about their surgery than the control group. Other oils such as sandalwood, neroli, and lavender have also been used in conventional medicine to help patients better manage anxiety.[37]

Certain essential oils have also been used by midwives to help reduce fear and anxiety during childbirth. A study in the *Journal of Alternative and Complementary Medicine* found that women who used aromatherapy during labor reported less pain overall and were able to use fewer pain medications.[38]

toxify the liver and gallbladder. This oil from a tropical tree in the Philippines can be used to improve mood, help release pent-up emotions like frustration, and act as an aphrodisiac.

Have fun experimenting. Revel in this "dirty" way of healing. And remember: different oils can be blended together to enhance their health benefits or can be blended with a base oil (such as coconut oil) for massages, shower gels, or body lotions. (See chapter 17 for some specific formulas.) The more comfortable you become with transitioning away from commercial, industrial products to homemade, essential-oil-based products, the more old friends you can welcome back into your gut and the greater ripple effect of health benefits you'll feel throughout your entire life.

— Gut Protectors: Healing Ourselves Naturally —

Our cavalier approach to antibiotics and other serious medication has brought us to a crossroads. We can either keep going down the path of chemical medicine and tempt an extremely serious fate . . . or we can recognize the folly of our ways, and reverse course. Move back to a simpler time, when we lived in harmony with our microbiome, and heal the body (and the gut) in a way that recognizes our connection to the Earth. The choice is ours.

▶ **Fewer pharmaceutical medicines** may reduce risk to the gut. Be diligent about potential risks, side effects, and alternatives. If you can find a nondrug alternative, please explore it—your gut will thank you!

▶ **Probiotics** are as effective as many mainstream drugs—but their side effects are significantly less devastating, if nonexistent. The upside is huge, the downside is negligible—the opposite outcome of 50 percent of the antibiotics used in this country.

▶ **Essential oils** are our original medicines—they healed us for millennia. It's high time we acknowledge their power and versatility, and return them to the place of respect they once held. Experiment with the different blends to find one that works for you.

We've covered the five ways that our guts have been devastated by modern life. Now, let's put all the solutions together into one integrated program, so you can begin to heal your gut and entire body.

10

The Eat Dirt Program

All health starts in the gut, and as you know by now, the chances are very good that your gut may be struggling with a leak. I've created a set of guidelines designed to help anyone get started today on repairing their leaky gut and getting back to optimal living. It's a simple five-step program:

1. Remove
2. Reseed
3. Restore
4. Release
5. Reseal

Once you have a week or two under your belt, you might turn to chapter 11, where you can further refine this program for your own specific gut type. A quiz will help you zero in on your core concerns, and your corresponding protocol will teach you which specific types of "dirt" (foods, supplements, and lifestyle practices) have proven the most beneficial to patients who share your type.

Many people find it helpful to start a notebook at the beginning of the Eat Dirt program. You can use your notebook any way you'd like— recording blood test results or shopping lists, or simply as a place to write your questions for yourself. At least for the first month or two, I would recommend using your notebook partially as a food journal that tracks your emotions and any physical symptoms in the same space. The objective here is to increase your awareness of your physical and emotional reactions to certain foods (or the removal of those foods!), so you can start to become more mindful about eating. I have found this practice allows my patients to explore the habits, tastes, and preferences that can drive our food choices—as well as help them become more conscious and less reactive about the choices they are making. Be sure to include notes about your digestive habits, how your skin looks and feels, what kinds of moods you're experiencing, or how your energy level changes—and generally how rested and fully satiated you feel. (If you're feeling ambitious, you might keep track of the shape, color, and frequency of your bowel movements, as they can give you—and your doctor—a tremendous amount of information about the health of your entire GI tract.)

First, let's review the Eat Dirt program's five steps that can restore healthy balance and welcome more beneficial microbes back into your personal microbiome.

TESTING YOUR SOIL

Are you curious about the diversity in your own gut? How will you know that these five core practices are working? Based on past experience with my patients, within two weeks you should certainly recognize changes in your digestive system, such as more frequent bowel movements. Greater energy is another sign that your inner soil is vibrant and dynamic.

But if you'd like to drill down to more detailed, specific information about your personal microbial balance, consider having your microbiome checked with a lab test. I've had good success with uBiome (www.ubiome .com) and recommend this biotech company to my patients. The stool sample is easy to do and costs eighty-nine dollars. Send a sample in, and a few weeks later you receive a lab report of all the bacterial comings and goings in your microbiome.

— Step 1: Remove —

As you might recall from chapter 5, the first step in the Eat Dirt program is to eliminate the foods that are damaging your health, such as gluten, processed foods, and dairy. You're officially on a mission to root out and eliminate all the antinutrients that are robbing your body of true nourishment. Go through your kitchen and throw out anything that appears on the list below. Half the reason people don't stick with healthier eating habits is the temptations sitting in their own pantries. Get out a garbage bag and remove these foods:

▶ **Wheat and other grains** contain antinutrients like gluten and lectin that can damage your intestinal lining and cause leaky gut. A 2013 European study found that wheat and other grains could increase chronic inflammation and risk of inflammation by triggering leaky gut and its resultant proinflammatory immune response.

▶ **Commercial cow's milk** is modified—through the pasteurization process—in ways that destroy vital enzymes and make lactose difficult to digest. According to a study published in the journal *Clinical and Experimental Immunology*, the processing of dairy alters the casein protein, creating a molecule that resembles gluten, which produces an inflammatory response.

▶ **Sugar** feeds the growth of bad bacteria and yeast, upsetting the balance and wreaking havoc on the digestive system. This causes certain microbes like staphylococcus and *H. pylori* to crowd out other beneficial bacteria and produce toxins themselves that damage the small intestine.

▶ **Hydrogenated oils**, including canola, soybean, corn, and vegetable oils, give rise to intestinal inflammation, which is both a cause and a result of leaky gut. These oils can be found in many supermarket products labeled as "natural." Salad dressings, condiments, soups, and snack chips are some of the most common sources of hydrogenated oils.

▶ **GMO foods**—produced from genetically modified plants like corn and soybeans—contain high levels of glyphosate, the active ingredient in the weed killer Roundup. My friend Jeffrey M. Smith, author of *Genetic Roulette*, reviewed a series of studies and found troubling research linking glyphosate and other components of GMOs to leaky gut, imbalanced gut bacteria, and damage to the intestinal wall.

▶ **Toxic chemicals**, commonly found in processed foods and beverages, destroy beneficial gut bacteria. Artificial sweeteners such as aspartame and sucralose alter the microbial composition in the gut. Pesticides, hormones, antibiotics, food colorings, and preservatives are among the most dangerous foods. Municipal tap water also exposes you to excess amounts of chlorine and fluoride, which have been linked to liver and intestinal damage.

THE EAT DIRT REPLACEMENT FOODS LIST

INSTEAD OF . . .	TRY . . .
Bread	ancient sprouted breads (made with amaranth, quinoa, buckwheat, spelt, or others) and paleo bread (made with coconut flour and almond flour)
Cereal	sprouted nut granola made from sprouted almonds, pecans, chia seeds, raisins, coconut flakes, cinnamon, raw honey, and sea salt
Cheesecake	homemade cashew cheesecake
Chips	kale chips from Alive and Radiant, sweet potato chips from Jackson's Honest Chips, and baked zucchini chips
Coffee (with sugar)	herbal tea or organic coffee with coconut creamer
Commercial meats	100 percent grass-fed organic beef, lamb, and venison, free-range poultry, nitrate-free turkey bacon, and organic beef sausage
Cookies and pastries	trail mix made with raisins, goji berries, cashews, almonds, coconut, and dark chocolate, and cookies and pastries made with coconut flour, almond flour, and raw honey
Crackers	Mary's Gone Crackers and Lydia's Grain-Free Crackers

INSTEAD OF . . .	TRY . . .
Dips	hummus, salsa, and guacamole
Energy bars	collagen bars, LäraBar bars with dates and nuts, or homemade protein bars
Energy drinks	coconut water, kombucha, or green tea with stevia
Farm-raised fish (such as Atlantic salmon and tilapia)	wild-caught salmon and other wild-caught fish such as halibut, tuna, sardines, and grouper
Fast food burger	bison burger on sprouted grain bun
French fries	baked sweet potato fries cooked in coconut oil and topped with sea salt, eggplant fries, and turnip fries
Fried chicken	Baked Artichoke Chicken (page 274)
Fruit juice or lemonade	strawberry lemonade made with 100 percent real strawberries and lemon juice, San Pellegrino sparkling water with lime juice, or coconut water
Ice cream	coconut ice cream or cashew ice cream
Lunch meat	grass-fed organic lunch meat, organic turkey, and grass-fed beef jerky
Mayonnaise	mixture of avocado, egg yolk, and apple cider vinegar
Microwave popcorn	stovetop popcorn or Pipcorn
Milk (cow's)	unsweetened coconut milk and unsweetened almond milk
Milk chocolate	organic dark chocolate (70 percent or more cocoa)
Milkshake	Hot Chocolate Smoothie (page 258)
Pastas	zucchini noodles, quinoa noodles, and Ezekiel 4:9 pasta
Peanut butter	sprouted almond and cashew butter from Blue Mountain Organics
Pizza	homemade pizza on sprouted tortilla
Processed cheese	raw cheeses from goat's milk and sheep's milk

(*continued on next page*)

INSTEAD OF . . .	TRY . . .
Refined oatmeal	chia seed pudding and sourdough sprouted oats, gluten-free
Salad dressing	olive oil, balsamic vinegar, hummus, coconut vinegar, and Bragg salad dressings and apple cider vinegar
High-sodium seasonings	sea salt, garlic, rosemary, turmeric, cilantro, basil, and black pepper
Soda (regular or diet)	strawberry lemonade with stevia, kombucha, coconut kefir, or herbal tea with stevia or raw honey
Sugar or artificial sweeteners	stevia, raw honey, dates, and cinnamon
Tortillas/wraps	lettuce, coconut wraps, and Ezekiel 4:9 tortillas and Ezekiel 4:9 sprouted corn tortillas
Vegetable oil and canola oil	coconut oil, olive oil, and ghee (clarified butter)
Whey protein powder	grass-fed whey protein powder, collagen protein powder, and sprouted vegan protein powder
White and wheat flour	coconut flour and almond flour
White or wheat bread	Ezekiel 4:9 bread or real sourdough
Yogurt or sour cream	goat's milk kefir and homemade yogurt

BONUS: For more healthy food swap ideas, check out the full-color replacement food list at www.draxe.com/replacement-food-list

— Step 2: Reseed —

Once you've eliminated the biggest offenders from your diet, your gut will get a little bit of a break. Now is a great time to bolster your beneficial bacteria by seeding your gut with microexposures of good guys.

These live bacteria, fungi, and yeasts are extremely helpful for keeping your gut healthy because they not only rally together with the commensals already in your gut, they actively reduce or prevent the growth of harmful bacteria in the digestive system.

A soil-based probiotic supplement is the most important supplement you can take to help repair leaky gut. (See chapters 6 and 9 for a full discussion.) Unfortunately, most probiotic supplements don't contain living soil-based organisms, so you will want to make sure you buy a brand that contains certain strains that have greater resistance and that are shelf stable. It's important to remember you need a large diversity of probiotic strains in your gut, because each organism serves a different purpose. Certain strains enhance immune function, others protect the intestinal lining from damage, and yet others destroy dangerous bacteria.

Also, don't forget to reseed your gut with good dirt in other ways, too:

▶ Spend time walking barefoot outside
▶ Shop at your local farmer's market for fresh produce

MOM'S CONSTIPATION RX

I mentioned earlier how my mother was able to "move things along" after many years of dealing with constipation. What really transformed her digestive tract was following my suggestion to go on the Budwig diet, which was developed by a German biochemist named Dr. Johanna Budwig in the 1950s.

The Budwig protocol is a popular natural health regime used to combat cancer and cellular disease. My mom consumed this drink every day as part of her holistic treatment. Here's the recipe (which she mixed in blender):

6 ounces goat's milk kefir (raw and organic)
3 tablespoons sprouted flax meal
2 tablespoons flaxseed oil
stevia to taste (optional)

My mother's chronic constipation soon disappeared because her digestion, detoxification, and overall gut health were rescued by this perfect combination of probiotic kefir and prebiotic flaxseed, along with gut-soothing flaxseed oil.

- ▶ Play with your dog or ride a horse
- ▶ Consume one tablespoon of raw local honey daily
- ▶ Dig in the soil of your garden
- ▶ Swim in the ocean and freshwater lakes
- ▶ Consume two servings daily of fermented foods
- ▶ Eat medicinal mushrooms like shiitake and green algae like spirulina

All of these opportunities for dirt microexposures help to continuously replenish and nourish the bacteria that are sloughed off each day, keeping them well fed and happy.

> **BONUS:** To download some gut-healing smoothie recipes, check out my bonus smoothie guide: www.draxe.com/smoothie-guide-bonus

— Step 3: Restore —

We did ourselves—and our guts—a grave disservice when we strayed from some of the traditional ways of growing, preparing, and eating food. Thankfully, changing these newer habits will also help reverse some of our modern health crises.

Restore your gut by eating the following foods:

- ▶ **Organic fruits, vegetables, meats, nuts, and other products.** The evidence is indisputable—we must strive to feed ourselves and our families organic as often as possible. While the prices may be a bit higher for these foods, the benefits far outweigh the costs. (And remember this dictum: pay either the farmer now, or the pharmacy later!) We can also take solace from the knowledge that these efforts are helping rebuild the soil for future generations.
- ▶ **Bone broth.** When they begin the restore phase of the Eat Dirt program, I recommend that my patients do a bone broth fast for three days, to give their leaky gut time to "reboot" and repair itself. The simmering process in making beef or chicken bone broth causes the bones and ligaments to release healing compounds like colla-

gen, proline, glycine, and glutamine, which have immune-boosting properties that help repair leaky gut.

The amino acids in bone broth that make up collagen and gelatin are critical gut-healing nutrients. These amino acids are used to repair the damaged intestinal lining and protect the gut from further damage, and are metabolic fuel for cells in the small intestine. A study conducted by the University of Nebraska Medical Center found that chicken soup (using homemade chicken broth) helped improve digestion, allergies, and asthma by improving immune function.

You can easily make your own bone broth. I have a great recipe for bone broth on page 255 in the Eat Dirt recipes chapter, where I share delicious recipes, each geared toward a particular gut type.

> **BONUS:** If you want some ideas for creating easy and great-tasting bone broth you can download my top ten bone broth recipes here: www.draxe .com/bone-broth-recipes-bonus

▶ **Raw cultured dairy.** Kefir, yogurt, and raw cheese contain high levels of vitamin B_{12}, calcium, magnesium, folate, enzymes, and probiotics. I would especially like to encourage you to try kefir, a creamy, tangy, and effervescent fermented milk beverage that's loaded with healthy microorganisms like *Lactobacillus acidophilus* and bifidobacteria.

I'm a big fan of traditional homemade yogurt (not store-bought versions), because the healthy bacteria that are generated during the production process greatly improve the microflora balance in the gut. There's a major difference between conventional dairy, like commercial milk and cheese, which can cause leaky gut, and organic cultured dairy and fermented goat's milk yogurt and kefir, which boast healthy fats and are teeming with beneficial bacteria.

▶ **Fermented vegetables.** Sauerkraut, pickled vegetables, and Asian examples like miso and kimchi are filled with fiber, digestion-enhancing enzymes, and beneficial bacteria. These traditional fermented foods are bursting with lactic acid bacteria that help balance the production of stomach acid.

▸ **Fermented beverages.** Apple cider vinegar (mixed with water), kvass, and kombucha are fermented beverages high in lactic and gluconic acids, as well as enzymes and probiotics that aid digestion.

▸ **Coconut products.** An array of coconut foods, including coconut oil, coconut flour, coconut milk, coconut butter, and coconut water, all benefit your gut. Coconut's medium-chain fatty acids are easier to digest than other fats, so they're better for those suffering from leaky gut (especially those with long-standing gallbladder issues). An all-star in this category is coconut kefir due to the high amount of probiotics that support a healthy digestive system.

Be sure to cook with coconut oil, which supports the immune system and can be used at all temperatures. Coconut oil contains lauric acid, known to reduce *Candida albicans*, fight bad bacteria, and create a hostile environment for viruses. Coconut oil has a way of absorbing fat-soluble vitamins, calcium, and magnesium while easing the strain on the pancreas. Medium-chain fatty acids are known for improving symptoms of gallbladder disease. A study published in *Antimicrobial Agents and Chemotherapy* found coconut oil's lauric acid and capric acid to be effective natural treatments for candida and yeast infections.[1]

DIY PROBIOTICS

I love the health benefits of kefir, yogurt, sauerkraut, kimchi, kombucha, and miso and appreciate how fermented foods like pickled carrots, beets, and cucumbers help tone and strengthen the immune system.

If you're a back-to-nature, DIY type of person, you can certainly make your own fermented foods and dairy products. Kefir is produced from raw milk that you can buy at a farmer's market, and you can make your own yogurt as long as you have the "starter" bacteria *Streptococcus thermophilus* and *Lactobacillus bulgaricus*. Kombucha, the fermented mushroom tea, can be produced in a large glass container on your kitchen counter. If you're interested in learning more about how to make your own fermented foods, you can go to my website, DrAxe.com.

BONUS: Want to know what to order, where to eat out, and how to travel and still heal leaky gut? Download my free bonus guide on how to heal leaky gut while on the go: www.draxe.com/eating-out-guide

▶ **Wild-caught salmon.** Ocean-caught fish are high in vitamin D, vitamin B$_{12}$, and omega-3 fatty acids. A study published in the *Journal of the American College of Nutrition* said that omega-3 fatty acids encourage the gut to cool off inflammation—as opposed to farmed fish, which have a higher ratio of proinflammatory omega-6s, which underscores the importance of eating wild-caught fish like salmon, mackerel, and cod.[2]

THE POWER OF PREBIOTICS

Prebiotics are foods and supplements that promote the health of beneficial microorganisms in the gut. We've talked about several different kinds throughout the book, including raw honey, medicinal mushrooms, and even blue-green algae like spirulina. However, one of the easiest ways to feed our good bugs is what our elders would've called "roughage"—good old-fashioned fiber.

This indigestible remnant of plant cells found in fruits, vegetables, whole grains, nuts, seeds, and beans comes in two types—soluble and insoluble—which can be thought of as "flush and scrub," respectively. Soluble fiber dissolves in water and moves through the digestive system to help with the elimination of toxins. That's the flushing side. Insoluble fiber, however, doesn't dissolve in water but works at scrubbing your digestive lining and also helps compel elimination. That's the scrubbing side.

Foods with a lot of soluble fiber cause us to chew thoroughly, slowing our eating and helping us to feel fuller and eat less. While soluble fiber slows digestion so that nutrients can be absorbed more evenly and slowly, its greater benefit is how soluble fiber detoxifies the digestive tract and kills off bad bacteria like candida.

(continued on next page)

With the foods below, you're front-loading your gut with nutrients that nourish the intestinal lining, provide fuel for the body, and help the liver's detoxification efforts. These attributes are why soluble fiber is a "fermentable fiber" that acts as a prebiotic, stimulating the growth of beneficial microbiota in the digestive tract. Aim to eat many kinds of vegetables, berries, and seeds so you get both soluble and insoluble fiber in proper ratios. (And don't forget: if you are adding fiber to your diet, be sure to drink more water to help move things through your body!)

Foods High in Prebiotic Soluble Fiber

apples	celery	oatmeal
artichokes	chia seeds	onions
asparagus	collards	pears
avocados	cucumbers	peas
beans	figs	pumpkin
blueberries	flaxseeds	raspberries
broccoli	garlic	sesame
brussels sprouts	hemp	spinach
cabbage	kale	strawberries
carrots	lentils	

BONUS: For the entire Leaky Gut Shopping List go to www.draxe.com/eat -dirt-shopping-list

Omega-3 fatty acids were also found to reduce the risk of inflammatory bowel disease and ulcerative colitis, according to a 2014 study performed by researchers at Leicester General Hospital in the United Kingdom. Anti-inflammatory omega-3 fats are also acquired when consuming grass-fed beef, lamb, wild game, walnuts, and certain seeds.[3]

▶ **Sprouted seeds and high-fiber foods.** Chia seeds, flaxseeds, and hemp seeds are great to add to smoothies, especially if they have been sprouted, which improves digestibility. Also, sprouted seeds are a superior source of fiber that acts as a prebiotic to feed and support the growth of beneficial bacteria. Don't forget steamed vegetables like broccoli, asparagus, and spinach, which feature specific types of fiber favored by good bugs. (Note: those with severe leaky gut may need to avoid seeds for a time, however, and consume cooked vegetables for fiber. Work with your doctor or nutritionist to determine the best diet for you.)

— Step 4: Release —

One of the biggest causes of leaky gut is emotional and mental stress. A 2014 study published in the journal *Gut* found that emotional or psychological stress greatly increased the risk of leaky gut and inflammatory bowel disease.[4] Here are six things you can do to reduce stress today and begin healing your gut:

Get a massage or reflexology treatment. It's easy for stress and tension to build up in your muscles, including your neck and shoulders. A nice relaxing massage or foot reflexology session has tremendous value at reducing stress. Moderate-pressure massage has been proven to reduce cortisol levels, relieve pain in fibromyalgia and rheumatoid arthritis, and improve the function of the parasympathetic nervous system. MRI studies have also shown that massage creates lasting changes in the brain in areas related to the stress response.[5]

Do something active. Hike a trail, ride a bike, go to an indoor rock climbing gym, or, if you have joint issues, get in a pool and do some water aerobics. Movement increases circulation, which naturally improves energy and also causes your body to release the "good mood hormones" known as endorphins.

Have a warm glass of chamomile tea in the evening to prepare your body for a restful night's sleep. Chamomile has the ability to relax the entire body and is a natural antispasmodic, which relieves tension in the neck, the shoulders, and even the gut. Recent research has also shown chamomile to reduce digestive spasms, such as stomachaches, and reduce symptoms of IBS.

Read something uplifting, whether it's your favorite novelist, an inspiring memoir, a self-help book, or a spiritual text. Wind down at the end of the day not by zoning out in front of the TV, but by engaging your mind in content that will boost your mood and help to unwind your stress.

Use essential oils of lavender, vetiver, roman chamomile, vanilla, orange, and ylang-ylang; try rubbing them on your neck and forehead. Also, you can buy a diffuser that you can leave running in your house all day and night. Essential oils contain therapeutic compounds that help relieve anxiety and improve mood. In a controlled study of sixty patients under stress while being treated in an intensive care unit, their nurses found that aromatherapy with essential oils increased the patients' quality of sleep and reduced their level of anxiety.[6]

Try a magnesium supplement to help relieve tense muscles and headaches. Take approximately five hundred milligrams a day and consume more magnesium-rich foods like avocado, pumpkin seeds, spinach, figs, and yogurt.

Listen to music for at least ten minutes a day. And if you want to drop your stress levels even further, sing! Singing allows your body to release deep-rooted stress, and according to a study published in the journal the *Gerontologist*, it can even improve memory, focus, and mood.[7]

Go "forest bathing." Go on a short walk in the woods, and take many deep breaths, consciously bringing the scent of the trees into your lungs. This form of aromatherapy is a practice called "shinrin-yoku," or "forest bathing," in Japanese. Researchers there have found breathing in the antimicrobial organic compounds called phytoncides—the woods' essential oils—decreased cortisol levels and blood pressure, enhanced immune system function, and stabilized nervous system activity.[8]

— Step 5: Reseal —

The final step of the Eat Dirt program is all about finishing what we set out to do—heal that leaky gut and use good, dirty practices to keep it closed as long as possible. First, try to avoid taking any unnecessary medications. If you're on a maintenance drug, or even on a short-term prescription that feels like it's not working the way you'd hope, seek out a naturopathic doctor or other health care provider to discuss your options.

Sometimes traditional Western doctors tend to just "fix it and forget it," writing out a prescription and sending you on your way. But you've seen how devastating drugs can be to the gut (and the entire body); before you accept your next prescription, perhaps take a moment to truly understand the mechanisms involved and the risks to other parts of the body. Supplements can be a nice Eat Dirt middle ground between foods and medicine—usually the results are a bit faster than those that come from food, but the potential risks and side effects are not nearly as dramatic as with medicine. Here are a few supplements that will help to reseal your gut:

- ▶ **Probiotics** are the most important part of resealing. A high-quality, live probiotic supplement will speed up the healing of the gut by restoring the balance of the bacteria. (See the very thorough discussion of probiotics in chapter 9.)
- ▶ **Digestive enzymes.** These nutrients completely break down proteins, fatty acids, complex sugars, and starches, which can reduce intestinal inflammation. Look for full-spectrum digestive enzyme supplements that contain:
  - ▶ protease, which breaks down proteins, including gluten
  - ▶ amylase, which breaks down starches
  - ▶ lipase, which breaks down fats
  - ▶ lactase, which breaks down lactose in dairy
- ▶ **L-glutamine.** Here's an essential amino acid with anti-inflammatory qualities as well as health benefits that include repairing the gut and intestinal lining. Another benefit of taking L-glutamine regularly is that it helps thicken cell walls and resist *Staphylococcus aureus* bacterial infections, according to a study published in *Antimicrobial Agents and Chemotherapy*. The highest quality is called l-alanyl-glutamine, which the intestines can use more readily.[9]
- ▶ **Licorice root.** One of my favorite adaptogenic herbs (meaning herbs that help your body adapt to stress), licorice root supports the adrenal glands by the way it aids gastric function and metabolism of cortisol, regulates carbohydrate metabolism and the immune system, and maintains blood pressure. Licorice root is especially beneficial for those dealing with leaky gut that's being exacerbated by emotional stress.
- ▶ **Collagen.** The secret behind bone broth's healing power is collagen, a protein that can be made into powder that gives skin, bone,

cartilage, and tendons their strength. Collagen contains the amino acids proline and glycine, which are essential building blocks to repair damaged intestinal lining. Supplementing with collagen protein powder can help restore the integrity and health of the mucosal lining.

▶ **Frankincense.** A 2015 study published in *PLoS ONE* found that frankincense (*Boswellia serrata*) protected the tight junctions of the gut from damage caused by inflammation.[10] Both frankincense essential oil and boswellia powder are effective remedies in treating leaky gut syndrome.

▶ **Other beneficial supplements.** Colostrum powder, slippery elm, aloe vera juice, chamomile, and the organic sulfur compound methylsulfonylmethane, or MSM, may help in healing leaky gut.

> **BONUS:** To see a more detailed list of the best supplements and herbs to heal leaky gut, check out this Top 25 Leaky Gut Supplement PDF: www .draxe.com/leaky-gut-supplements-bonus

I've been amazed at the extent of the total body transformation my patients can experience, if they're willing to commit to the Eat Dirt program for a couple of months. My highest hope for you, as you move forward with the Eat Dirt philosophy, would be for you to become more conscious of each aspect of your health, and how your activities, habits, choices, and beliefs, and all the systems in your body and your life, interconnect with each other to determine the course of your life.

You've reached the end of the Eat Dirt foundational program. I hope these steps have begun to create real change in your health. However, if you believe you still have a larger health issue you'd like to tackle, or if you simply want to optimize your results, you can take the Eat Dirt approach one step further and investigate your specific gut type. In the next chapter, I'll share the story behind the birth of the gut types, which coincided with the realization that I needed to learn how to take my own advice!

part three

HEAL FOR YOUR GUT TYPE

11

Healing the Whole Body

At this point in our journey, we've thoroughly discussed leaky gut—how it develops, how we make it worse, and how we can begin to make it better. By now I hope you've started to implement some of the Eat Dirt program principles in your life, such as eating more organic produce and fermented foods, managing your stress, and getting outside more often. But what if you're still suffering from digestive distress, feeling fatigued, or holding on to excess weight? What if your gut issues don't seem to be fully resolved?

We know that the body's organs and systems are inextricably linked—the health of each is dependent upon, and affects, all others. When it comes to leaky gut, multiple systems throughout the body are involved. Following every thread of this delicate web is part of the diagnostic process that helps us identify leaky gut. Once we have that diagnosis, we can turn our attention back to the web that created it and address each individual thread in our treatment.

Treating thousands of patients over the years, I've seen firsthand how unique every person's health story really is. For some, the root cause of their leaky gut might be candida overgrowth. For others, it might be immune system dysfunction. When specific body systems are not functioning optimally, the path may require a slightly different approach to healing. If you can zero in on what's going awry in your body and identify the weakest link, you can begin to fix systemic problems at their source.

If you've been helped by the basic Eat Dirt plan, that's wonderful. But if you find that you need a bit more help, or you want to customize your plan even further, you may want to learn more about the five leaky gut types. At the end of this chapter, you will find a small excerpt from the Eat Dirt gut type quiz; the full quiz is hosted on my website (www.draxe.com/gut-type-quiz). This quiz can help you to determine which gut type best reflects your situation. Once you have your gut type, you can turn to the corresponding chapter in part 3 to refine your core plan with some type-specific modifications. If you've been hoping for more dramatic results, you may find these specific guidelines are just what you need.

These types hold personal resonance for me, because I discovered my own at a time when my health was at an all-time low. Early in my career, when I was starting to help many people to heal from leaky gut, I still hadn't truly connected all the dots about this mysterious condition nor refined the nuances until I experienced it for myself. (Hey, we all need a little help sometimes!)

— Doctor, Heal Thyself —

Before I started my clinical practice, I did a six-month internship in Naples, Florida, which necessitated a short-term house rental. Toward the end of my internship, I developed digestive issues and a red flushing on my face. I also noticed that whenever I ate certain foods, such as eggs and dairy products, my nose would start to run. I had never experienced anything like this and wasn't completely sure what was causing my symptoms.

Just before I left Naples, I was replacing an air filter inside my rental home when I found mold in the air duct. I determined that mold toxicity was the probable cause of my skin inflammation as well as the digestive issues and food sensitivities I'd been experiencing. A couple of weeks later, I moved to Nashville to open my wellness clinic, which turned out to be the busiest time of my life.

I worked six days a week, typically putting in twelve-hour days. Not only was my clinic expanding—it would quickly grow into one of the largest functional medicine clinics in the country—I was also training for triathlons before work or during the middle of the day, taking two-hour blocks to swim, run, and ride my bike.

In the midst of this physically demanding and stressful period, I continued to have skin inflammation as well as sensitivities to a variety of foods. I was determined to find out why my body hadn't completely rebounded from the mold exposure, so I ordered a series of tests for myself:

- an Organic Acids Test (OAT), which revealed that I had vitamin and mineral deficiencies for vitamin B_{12}, zinc, and iron
- an IgG test and an IgE test, which both showed food sensitivities and food allergies
- a stool test, which told me that I had an imbalance of good and bad microbes in the gut, notably an excess of yeast and a lactobacillus probiotic deficiency

The findings surprised me—I'd always considered myself exceptionally healthy, my diet rich in organic foods. In response to the four tests, though, I began taking digestive enzymes and probiotics, and beginning each day with a bowl of homemade bone broth—the nutrient-dense, glutamine-and-collagen-rich consommé we talked about in chapter 6 that supports gut health.

I'd say that over the next year, I got 70 percent better. The red flaking skin improved dramatically, but my health issues still weren't completely resolved. I knew I was missing something that would restore my gut health back to 100 percent.

Motivated to find answers, I went online to some of my favorite medical resources. I came across a journal article that discussed the benefits of traditional Chinese medicine (TCM) in dealing with similar symptoms. Intrigued, I contacted a colleague who was formally trained in this field, Dr. Gil Ben-Ami, an Israeli-born acupuncturist and herbalist.

I consulted with Dr. Gil to better understand the essential teachings of Chinese medicine. Along with many other fascinating details, Dr. Gil explained that two of the favored diagnostic tools in TCM were examining the tongue and feeling the pulse. Later that day, I went home and noticed that my tongue had redness and indentations along the edges. I soon learned that this was a sign of heat and stagnation in my liver and gallbladder.

My medical training had taught me that when the liver is stressed, fats are not digested properly, which stresses the small intestine and ultimately causes gut permeability. I researched foods that best support liver function and discovered that sour and bitter foods were among the most nourishing, as well as foods that were green and "living"—salads, sprouts, green apples. This process also helped me focus on a very important issue: I realized I had to do something about the stress in my life, especially my long work hours. In Chinese medicine, stress is the root cause of all disease and is just as important as—if not more important than—diet.

I prescribed myself a plan to reduce stress, which included taking Saturdays and Sundays completely off, even silencing my smartphone. (I'll admit that was hard.) I scheduled more free time during the work-week and even started reading some novels for fun, something I hadn't done since English classes in college.

After thirty days, most of my symptoms disappeared, and within three months, I felt as though I had completely healed and recovered from leaky gut.

My personal experience with leaky gut really helped me to understand what my patients were going through—I could definitely empathize with their frustrations! I also knew it was time to put my newfound knowledge to work, to further refine the Eat Dirt program to work for more resistant or tricky cases, like mine.

— Marrying East with West —

The more I studied Chinese medicine, the more I learned about how to look at illness as a matter of disharmony and imbalance rather than something to be solved with drugs. Eastern medicine has developed over thousands of years, based on individualized research, with millions of case studies. Something about this highly specific approach felt more genuine and helpful to me—and more reflective of my own approach—than the current iteration of Western medicine.

Modern Western medicine tends to compartmentalize bodily systems, viewing the digestion process as separate and distinct from other processes. When we experience digestive issues, most physicians or specialists will try to "fix" the ailment—or the organ—with prescription drugs. But in TCM, every system is viewed as connected to—and influencing—the other. And good digestion is considered to be central to good health. Zhang Jie Bin, known as one of the four great masters from the Ming dynasty, wrote, "The doctor who wants to nourish life has to tonify the stomach and spleen."[1]

Chinese medicine holds that the body is composed of five elements (also known as five phases): wood, fire, earth, metal, and water. Every person is a unique and characteristic blend of the influences of all these elements. When I first read about the five elements, I thought, *Is this a little too "out there" for me?* But as I continued to uncover case studies and study the core principles, I began to identify very clear correlations between the five phases and some of the most common patterns I see in my own practice.

In TCM, each phase is connected to the health of certain organs in the body, specific colors, one of the five senses, a season of the year, and certain emotions. Each element helps us understand how structures and systems in our bodies are interdependent.

- ▶ **Wood** is related to the liver and gallbladder, likes the color green and sour foods, is associated with spring, and has frustration and anger as emotions.
- ▶ **Fire** is related to the heart, small intestines, and nervous system, likes the color red and bitter foods, is associated with summer, and has fear and joy as emotions.
- ▶ **Earth** is related to the stomach, spleen, and pancreas, likes the color yellow and sweet foods, is associated with late summer, and has pensiveness as an emotion.
- ▶ **Metal** is related to the lungs and large intestines, likes the color white and pungent foods, is associated with autumn, and has sadness as an emotion.

▶ **Water** is related to the kidneys and bladder, likes the color black and salty foods, is associated with winter, and has fear as an emotion.

In many ways, the five elements are similar to the Myers-Briggs Type Indicator or the DISC profile tests, developed in the last century to assess personality types. All of these approaches were developed after many years (or centuries, in the case of TCM) of careful study and pattern recognition.

After reading various TCM assessment tools, I identified most closely with the wood element, which is related to liver and gallbladder function, affecting the tendons, ligaments, and neck. Learning that those with a wood element liked sour foods was interesting. Even as a young kid walking into a fast food restaurant with my family, I *loved* pickles on my hamburger. And ever since I embraced a healthier way of eating, I've gravitated toward tart-tasting kefir, sauerkraut, and apple cider vinegar mixed with water. I also liked sprouts, peas, arugula, and green apples—foods that are vivid green in color (and green has always been one of my favorite colors!).

In the wood element, the liver and the gallbladder are paired as yin and yang organs—two halves that, when put together, demonstrate wholeness. These organs work together to produce and store secretions that digest fats.

I discovered that TCM dovetailed nicely with my own approach to healing leaky gut and complemented everything I'd learned in Western and functional medicine—yet held out the promise of a new dimension to understand. It was through studying the principles of TCM that I formulated the five gut types. I was excited and intrigued to see how defining the five gut types helped me to carefully articulate disparate aspects of my patients' health that I'd never been able to understand before. Suddenly, I not only had a central, unifying frame of reference for my patients' struggles with leaky gut; I had more specific and nuanced dietary and lifestyle recommendations for each of them.

— The Five Gut Types —

Read through the following list to see if any of the gut types seem similar to your individual health status. Do you see yourself in any of these descriptions?

- **Candida gut**, related to yeast overgrowth, is often caused by birth control pills and a diet high in sugar and foods that cause "dampness," such as cow's milk dairy, bananas, and wheat. Candida gut is related to the earth and fire elements in Chinese medicine.
- **Stressed gut** happens when emotional stress, excess sugar, and carbohydrate consumption stress the adrenals, kidneys, and thyroid, which then cause leaky gut. Stressed gut is related to the water element in Chinese medicine.
- **Immune gut** is triggered by taking prescription antibiotics and medications, consuming a diet high in inflammatory foods, and going through emotions of grief, depression, and disappointment. These issues can cause weakened immunity, food sensitivities, and inflammatory bowel disease. Immune gut is related to the metal element in Chinese medicine.
- **Gastric gut** comes from chronically poor digestion, antacids, and a lack of nutrient absorption that prevents the gut from maintaining healthy organs, which often results in small intestinal bacterial overgrowth (SIBO), acid reflux, bloating, or gas. Gastric gut is related to the fire and earth elements in Chinese medicine.
- **Toxic gut** develops when a diet high in bad fats and toxins overworks the liver and gallbladder, and often results in toxicity, gallbladder disease, and skin issues. Toxic gut is related to the wood element in Chinese medicine.

Does any one gut type immediately leap out at you? Normally people get a "gut reaction" (ha!) to the one that fits them best. To help you further determine your particular gut type, please go to www.draxe.com /gut-type-quiz. (The logarithm of the online quiz is much more sophisticated than I could duplicate here within the book, so I suggest you use that tool.) Here's a preview of a few of the questions asked in the quiz.

— Gut Type Quiz Preview —

The answers to questions such as these, both individually and in combination with one another, will help the Gut Type Quiz to zero in on your specific gut type. (While this sample will not help you diagnose your type, it can help you see the wide range of symptoms and signals that may be related to leaky gut.)

1. Do you have cravings for sugar or baked goods?
2. Do you have any food allergies or food sensitivities?
3. Have you ever had candida or any yeast, parasites, or fungal overgrowth?
4. Do you suffer from digestive issues like diarrhea, constipation, or inflammatory bowel disease?
5. Do you have gallstones, liver issues, or any health problems with your gallbladder?
6. Do you experience bloating or gas after meals on a regular basis?
7. What are the biggest emotions you experience when something doesn't go your way or you face adversity?

   ▸ overwhelmed/stressed/exhausted
   ▸ upset/depressed
   ▸ anxiousness/worry
   ▸ nervousness/emotionally charged
   ▸ frustration/anger

8. Do you have hormonal imbalances such as a thyroid issue or have such a slow metabolism that you can't lose weight?
9. Have you ever been diagnosed with or suspected that you have an autoimmune disease such as Hashimoto's, celiac, gastritis, chronic fatigue syndrome, fibromyalgia, or multiple sclerosis?

10. Have you ever been exposed to any toxins that have caused health issues for you?

11. Do you have any heart-related issues such as high cholesterol or high blood pressure?

12. Do you normally have a white coating on your tongue after consuming carbohydrates?

13. Do you feel tired or exhausted, even when you get enough sleep, or have adrenal fatigue?

14. Do you experience indigestion, small intestinal bacterial overgrowth (SIBO), or acid reflux more than once a week?

15. Do you regularly experience a moderate to high level of emotional stress?

16. Do you have skin complaints such as red skin, dry skin, acne, eczema, or psoriasis?

Remember: To get answers on your specific gut type, take the more in-depth version of this quiz at www.draxe.com/gut-type-quiz. You'll get a full-color printout and recommendations, as well as learn your secondary gut type.

The goal of the Gut Type Quiz is to help you clarify the possible symptoms you're experiencing and what organs are affected. Please know that the quiz is a guide, not an absolute. The questions were designed to help you focus on a particular protocol of foods that will nourish any specific organ weaknesses and help you overcome your body's version of leaky gut. If you have a strong sense that you may be a different gut type, feel free to follow that gut type's plan. (Also, while most of us have one dominant gut type, you may find upon repeating the quiz that you have a secondary gut type. If so, you'll want to support that as well; feel free to combine the recommendations of both types in a way that makes sense for your life and preferences.)

In the following five chapters, I have created customized protocols for each gut type. While I recommend that everyone starts with the core Eat Dirt program, if you find that you're not getting the results that you'd hoped for, or if you simply want to enhance your results, these personalized diet, supplement, and lifestyle plans can help you heal your specific root cause of leaky gut.

Before you flip to the chapter corresponding to your gut type, here are a few things to consider:

1. **The Gut Type Quiz tells you what you likely are, but it's important to listen to your body.** Pay attention to how you feel after you eat, and note which foods make you feel good, and which foods seem to be a problem. I recommend starting a food journal to track your reaction to different foods and supplements.

2. **Your results could change over time as you improve or face different stressors in the future.** The body is constantly reacting and changing, so it's possible to be one gut type now, but a different gut type a year from now when you're under a new type of stress. As the body changes, you need to change your protocol to support specific organ systems in a different way.

3. **Be aware that emotions cause organ dysfunction.** Everyone experiences multiple emotions daily, but if you've recently experienced a major trauma—a death in the family, a serious accident, getting laid off at work—it's not surprising that you could be experiencing leaky gut. Focus your efforts on relaxation and stress relief first, and be patient with yourself—it may take some time for your body to rebound.

So, are you ready to get started? If you know your gut type, go ahead and jump to the chapter that corresponds to that type, review the recommendations, and begin making additional changes in the foods you eat, the supplements you take, and the lifestyle you lead. As you heal your leaky gut, you will likely begin to experience a vast improvement in your health, on many levels.

12

Healing Candida Gut

THE CANDIDA GUT TYPE PRESCRIPTION

Causes	A high-sugar diet, antibiotics, and chronic anxiety.
The Right Diet	Low in sugar, high in probiotics.
The Right Supplements	Probiotics, oil of oregano, and pau d'arco tea.
Good Practices	Avoid white and brown sugar, coffee, alcohol, and grains.

Candida gut starts with *Candida albicans*, the most common type of yeast infection found in the mouth, intestinal tract, and vagina; it often affects the gut, skin, and other mucous membranes. When you have an overgrowth of yeast in the body, certain types of bacteria and yeast produce toxins that degrade the tight junctions inside the intestinal lining, causing leaky gut. If you could see yeast in a petri dish, you'd immediately notice that it has long roots (called plural hyphae). At the advanced stages of a *Candida albicans* yeast infection, these fungal branches spread along the gut wall, literally pulling cells apart.[1]

Candida gut is also related to dampness in the body, a traditional Chinese medicine concept in which there's a pathological accumulation of fluids in the body. Candida, as a fungal infection, flourishes in a damp environment, and dampness in the digestive tract is one of the prime causes of candida gut. The chief sign of candida gut is having a white coating on the tongue. A runny nose and coughing up phlegm are also manifestations of dampness. Dampness can also occur in the gut, which is exhibited by weight gain, slow metabolism, and loose stools. The top two foods that produce dampness are dairy products and foods with refined sugar. Wheat can be another big producer of dampness.

Regular consumption of damp foods can weaken the digestive system and undermine optimal health, especially if you live in a damp climate. The three organs that come under the most stress from this type of diet are the spleen, pancreas, and small intestine because of candida's chameleon-like ability to change from a noninvasive, sugar-fermenting yeast into a fungus that produces those long, rootlike structures that penetrate the intestinal wall.

Causes of candida overgrowth include the following:

- long courses of antibiotics
- birth control pills
- sugary foods and refined grains
- dairy
- cold foods
- diabetes
- cancer treatments
- negative emotions

Unlike antibiotics, birth control pills do not directly cause a yeast infection or candida overgrowth syndrome, but when combined with a diet high in sugary foods, birth control pills can adversely affect the body and produce a candida infection. Some women find that birth control pills instigate yeast infections, even long after the initial candida infection is gone.

Sugar feeds the growth of candida yeast and bad bacteria. Those with type 1 or type 2 diabetes have raised sugar levels in the body, so those with diabetes are at greater risk. Remember, refined grains immediately break down into sugars that feed yeast and contribute to fungal overgrowth. The worst foods with refined grains are pretzels, crackers, dry cereals, foods with enriched white flour, and beer. Gluten can accelerate candida gut, especially in those with preexisting sensitivity to gluten. Milk, cheese, and cream contain lactose, a simple sugar that provides fuel for candida. Kefir and yogurt are better, because most of the lactose disappears during the fermentation process.

According to Chinese medicine, different emotions impact specific organs. For example, the spleen and stomach are most affected by high levels of anxiety and worry, which increases susceptibility to candida.

Warning signs for candida gut include:

- exhaustion and extreme fatigue
- food sensitivities
- cravings for sweets
- bad breath
- white coating on the tongue
- brain fog (lack of focus, poor physical coordination, difficulty staying on task, poor memory)
- hormone imbalance (estrogen dominance)
- joint pain
- loss of sex drive
- chronic sinus and allergy issues
- gas and bloating
- urinary tract infections

— The Candida Gut Type Action Plan —

For those with candida gut, their good-to-bad bacteria ratio is unbalanced. Once harmful bacteria rise above the 15 percent mark, they can slow down or stop the immune system from working properly and set off a chain reaction that promotes disease, interferes with the proper digestion of food and absorption of nutrients, and even adversely influences gene activity.

It's important to eliminate candida overgrowth as soon as possible, because when the immune system is not performing properly, a candida infection can migrate to other areas of the body, including membranes around the heart. In order to clear candida from your body and heal leaky gut, you must begin supporting your small intestine and spleen with a better diet and lifestyle.

According to Chinese medicine, cold foods are hard on your spleen, one of the chief organs for producing red blood cells. Most people would think that sipping smoothies and cold vegetable juice and eating lots of salads made with healthy vegetables are good for the body—and they can be—but not when you have candida gut. You want to be consuming warm beverages such as tea and smoothies made from room-temperature ingredients.

An example of an ideal meal for candida gut would be warm bone broth soup, a helping of warmed-up fermented vegetables like sauerkraut or kimchi, and drinking a warm tea. Adding spaghetti squash or butternut squash to your bone broth soup can help you overcome sugar cravings common with candida gut. Pau d'arco tea, sweetened with stevia, can improve the function of the spleen and help clear out candida from your system. I recommend two or three cups of pau d'arco tea a day to my patients with candida gut.

The more bitter foods you eat, the better. Shop for kale, blueberries, and cranberries. Sour foods like kefir and yogurt are fantastic for candida gut. For dessert, bake an apple in the oven and use that to make a smoothie with cinnamon, collagen powder, and room-temperature coconut milk.

— Your Four-Step Strategy for Healing Candida Gut —

Review the explanations of candida gut and continue to educate yourself on what causes candida and its symptoms. Then follow the natural treatments in this section. Also, as you go, keep an eye on your tongue to see if the white coating is lessening—that can be a good indicator of how you're improving.

1. Eliminate Triggers: Foods Toxic to the Small Intestine and Spleen

- ▸ Avoid gluten and processed grains, and any foods and beverages with sugar.
- ▸ Avoid caffeine, which stimulates digestion so that food passes through the small intestine too quickly without its nutrients being absorbed. Caffeine also increases the heart

rate, which is significant, since cardiovascular problems are common for people with candida gut.

▶ Avoid alcohol, which is basically sugar and known to quickly increase yeast and fungal infections.

▶ Remove foods that cause dampness: milk, ice cream, cheese, eggs, sugar, artificial sweeteners, wheat, breads, pastas, refined flours, tofu, fatty meats like pork bacon, fruit juice, coffee, beer, fried foods, peanuts, nut butters, bananas, raw fruit, and soy milk.

2. Consume Therapeutic Foods

▶ Bitter foods are among the most therapeutic foods for the small intestine.

▶ Warm starchy vegetables in small amounts, according to ancient Chinese medicine, support the spleen in clearing candida from the body. Warming fall vegetables include sweet potatoes, yams, peas, mung beans, lentils, kidney beans, adzuki beans, carrots, beets, corn, butternut squash, spaghetti squash, acorn squash, zucchini, yellow squash, rutabaga, and pumpkin. You don't want to go overboard on these foods because they do contain moderate levels of carbohydrates. Aim for about two to three servings earlier in the day.

At night, consume less starch and mostly nonstarchy vegetables, broth, and organic meat.

▶ Fermented vegetables such as sauerkraut and kimchi replenish the good bacteria needed to control yeast and help rebuild the good bacteria in your gut.

▶ Organic meats such as grass-fed beef, lamb, venison, chicken, duck, turkey, wild game, wild-caught fish, chicken liver, and beef liver are superior protein sources. Don't forget that beef bone broth is greatly beneficial.

▶ Warm soups made in a slow cooker with nonstarchy vegetables like broccoli, cauliflower, cabbage, kale, and chard are recommended.

▶ In the nuts and seeds arena, stick with small servings. Ground flaxseeds, chia seeds, and pumpkin seeds support healthy blood sugar and contain zinc and omega-3 fatty acids.

▶ Cook with coconut oil and use olive oil in your salad dressings. Both contain antimicrobials and antioxidants that can halt candida growth.

▶ Stevia is your best option for sweetening your teas, since it doesn't contain sugar. Another option is a small amount (one teaspoon) of manuka honey.

▶ Recommended herbal teas are pau d'arco, chai, and licorice.

▶ Replace ice water with warm tea during meals.

3. Treat with Supplements

▶ Look for nutritional supplements with probiotics, which keep the good bacteria strong in the gut.

▶ Take natural antifungals or antiyeast products. Oregano oil, hemicellulose, berberine, caprylic acid, and thyme essential oil are superior sources and give great results.

▶ To support the spleen, look for supplements that contain herbs such as gentian, ginseng, skullcap, coptis, gardenia, and licorice.

▶ Try selenium, which relieves oxidative stress.

▶ Garlic kills fungus and boosts the immune system.

▶ Grapefruit seed extract powerfully reduces candida.

4. Transform Your Lifestyle

▶ According to ancient Chinese medicine, those who experience candida gut tend to have emotional responses like worrying, feeling anxious, and obsessing over everything. Work on reducing stress in your life. A good place to start is by spending time with close friends.

▶ Set boundaries. A great book that teaches you how to do that is *Boundaries: When to Say Yes, How to Say No*, by Henry Cloud and John Townsend. Read that book and start setting boundaries in your life.

▶ The next time you're inclined to push yourself beyond your physical abilities, remind yourself how you end up feeling exhausted. Try saying no the next time you're asked to help at the next community event, for example.

- This is a good time to declutter your life, your house, and your responsibilities. Get out a sheet of paper and write down all the good things and great things you're doing in life. Then concentrate on the great things.
- Those with candida gut are known for their empathy and strong feelings of responsibility. But you can't fix the world. Learn what your limitations are. Stop worrying about another person or situation that you can't do anything about anyway.
- At the same time, don't wall yourself away from the world. Company and conversation can be quite therapeutic, especially if your friend has a listening ear.
- Clear your mind. Meditate, pray, or sit still on a comfortable couch at least once a day. Step out into nature and take time to smell the roses. Even routine tasks like gardening and raking leaves can help in unexpected ways.
- Lighten things up . . . watch one of your favorite romantic comedies, read a fun book, or work on organizing your digital photos.
- Try acupuncture therapy, a great natural treatment for candida gut. Specific types of needling support the spleen and small intestine. Acupuncture has been used for thousands of years to treat candida symptoms and strengthen the spleen.
- Take a healing bath using essential oils like oregano, clove, and myrrh, which can reduce the growth of microbes and fungi. You can also rub them onto your skin.

— Candida Gut Daily Routine —

7:00 a.m. Upon Waking

Take ten to twenty minutes and read an uplifting spiritual book.

8:00 a.m. Breakfast and Supplements

Enjoy a low-sugar, gut-friendly breakfast. Pack your lunch and snacks (if you didn't the night before) and take your first round of supplements of probiotics and herbal remedies.

12:00 p.m. Lunch
Lunch can be light, but be sure to include some warm vegetables and organic meat.

3:00 p.m. Herbal Tea
Drink an eight-to-sixteen-ounce glass of warm herbal tea. Pau d'arco tea is the best and is effective for supporting the spleen.

5:00 p.m. Get Active
Do a fun workout in a group setting like barre, Pilates, or burst training. Or go on a bike ride or a brisk walk through the neighborhood.

6:00 p.m. Dinner and Supplements
Be sure your dinner includes several servings of warm vegetables and organic meat.

Take your supplements of probiotics and herbal remedies.

8:00 p.m. Massage or Journaling Before Bedtime
Have your partner give you a massage or do some journaling. You could also take a healing bath with Epsom salts and lavender oil to relax your body.

10:00 or 10:30 p.m. Bedtime
Meditate quietly and introspectively. Resist the temptation to get on social networks or embark on a late outing with friends. Wind down or read an uplifting book and get some quality rest.

— Candida Gut Nourishing Foods List —

Meat/Protein (three-to-five-ounce servings)
- kefir (raw, organic)
- yogurt (goat's milk and cultured for twenty-four hours or longer)
- wild-caught fish
- lamb
- bison
- lean beef
- venison
- turkey
- bone broth
- collagen powder (bone broth in powder form)

Vegetables (cooked)

- asparagus
- broccoli
- butternut squash
- carrots
- cauliflower
- celery
- chard
- garlic
- kale
- kimchi
- onions
- pumpkin
- sauerkraut
- spaghetti squash
- spinach
- turnips
- yellow squash
- zucchini

Fruits (one serving daily maximum)

- blueberries
- cranberries
- green apples
- lemon
- lime

Grains (sprouted)

- amaranth
- Job's Tears barley
- quinoa
- corn

Legumes

- adzuki beans
- red lentils

Fats/Oils

- coconut oil
- olive oil
- flaxseed oil

Flours

- coconut flour

Herbs

- cardamom
- cinnamon
- cloves
- ginseng
- parsley
- turmeric
- thyme
- oregano

Sweeteners

- manuka honey (one teaspoon)
- stevia

Beverages

- room-temperature water with lemon
- herbal teas

Seeds/Nuts (one-tablespoon serving)

- chia seeds
- flaxseeds
- hemp seeds
- pumpkin seeds

Danger Foods

- dairy
- products with yeast (like breads)
- raw foods
- refined grains
- sugar

13

Healing Stressed Gut

THE STRESSED GUT TYPE PRESCRIPTION

Causes	Emotional stress, thyroid issues, adrenal fatigue, and high cortisol levels.
The Right Diet	A diet high in nutrient-dense foods and low in sugar.
The Right Supplements	Vitamin B_{12}, selenium, and adaptogenic herbs such as licorice root and ashwagandha.
Good Practices	Learning to let go of stress in your life.

Did you know that the bacteria in your body can tell when you're stressed out? If you're frustrated by a traffic jam, worried about a loved one, or building up tension in a busy day, your body releases a pair of stress hormones: cortisol and epinephrine. These hormones not only halt the growth of beneficial bacteria and cause microbiome-disrupting yeast to proliferate, they're a direct cause of leaky gut. Mental strain and anxiety can also wear down your kidneys, adrenal glands, and thyroid, which can affect every hormone in your body.

With stressed gut, a stressful mental state triggers leaky gut syndrome, with symptoms that include:

▶ impaired absorption of nutrients
▶ reduced oxygen to the organs

▶ less blood flow to the digestive tract—four times less
▶ fewer enzymes in the gut—up to twenty thousand times fewer!

A pair of thumb-sized organs located just above the kidneys, the adrenal glands aid in the production of more than fifty hormones that drive almost every bodily function. Each adrenal gland is made up of two distinct structures; the outer part of the adrenal glands is called the adrenal cortex while the inner region is known as the adrenal medulla. The hormones produced by the adrenal cortex are necessary for life— they affect every function, organ, and tissue in the body. In contrast, the adrenal medulla secretes the hormones epinephrine and norepinephrine, in direct correlation to the level of stress you're undergoing.

You may know epinephrine by its other name, adrenaline. When you're under stress or suddenly find yourself in a fight-or-flight situation, the adrenal medulla produces epinephrine, which increases blood sugar (for immediate energy) and drives blood to the muscles and the brain (for increased responsiveness). Norepinephrine causes narrowing of the blood vessels, resulting in increased blood pressure. The adrenal cortex releases corticosteroids (including cortisol) to regulate blood pressure, increase cardiovascular function, manage the immune response, and suppress inflammatory reactions. When we're also experiencing leaky gut, the adrenal glands do their best to cope with the inflammatory response and struggle to keep up. Unfortunately, it's mostly a losing battle. Then the kidneys, spleen, and thyroid can become overloaded. In response, the immune system produces antibodies that damage thyroid cells and interfere with the thyroid's ability to make key hormones. This can lead to Hashimoto's disease, an autoimmune thyroid condition that is responsible for 90 percent of thyroid disease today.

People whose primary emotional responses to conflict are fear, indecisiveness, or uncertainty tend to have symptoms of stressed gut. Those who are known for their strong will, uncompromising determination, or for exercising caution when approaching situations or people can be prone as well. Stressed gut types are deep thinkers, constantly analyzing every angle of a situation to determine the best course of action.

Many with stressed gut are type-A personalities and achievement minded. When adversity strikes, however, they can become hermitlike and turn into workaholics who can't switch off when it's quitting time. They are the ones still answering emails after dinner and still working on reports and presentations right up until they drop their exhausted bodies into bed. Similarly, many with stressed gut value family, friends, and remaining in contact with people, thus creating a push-pull tension: someone who's become a solitary worker but also wants to be with people.

The challenge for stressed gut people is to put fear and indecisiveness in their place while fully expressing creativity in life. For those who can't meet that challenge, they inadvertently put stress on their adrenals, kidneys, and thyroid glands, leading to digestive issues and leaky gut. It's not uncommon for stressed gut people to also experience urinary issues, low libido, infertility, and other hormone-related problems.

Stress from heartbreak and gut-wrenching events like the death of a loved one, a divorce, or serious surgery lead to stressed gut. Prolonged stress from financial hardships, bad relationships, and fear of being laid off at work increase tension inside the gut. These issues are very real. At the end of the day, stressed gut flows out of emotional turmoil, especially difficulties that get internalized and produce feelings of being stressed out.

When the adrenal glands can't cope any longer, adrenal fatigue sets in. Adrenal fatigue can affect other organs like the small intestine and spleen and eventually lead to nutrient malabsorption. When the adrenal glands stop producing hormones efficiently, every bodily function is affected and you could experience symptoms like:

- ▶ morning fatigue or trouble waking up
- ▶ decreased libido
- ▶ depression
- ▶ muscle weakness
- ▶ poor focus
- ▶ bone loss
- ▶ inflammation
- ▶ increased allergies
- ▶ difficulty sleeping
- ▶ fatigue

- ► cravings for sugar
- ► thinning hair or hair loss
- ► weight gain
- ► muscle tension

If you're experiencing any of these adrenal fatigue side effects, then you're likely dealing with stressed gut.

— The Stressed Gut Type Action Plan —

With stressed gut, the first and most important things you need to address are diet and lifestyle. Two of the worst dietary triggers of stressed gut are caffeine and alcohol.

Caffeine interferes with your sleep cycle and makes it difficult for your adrenal glands to recover from the lack of full rest. If you must drink coffee or a caffeinated beverage, then one small serving before noon is less harmful.

Try drinking herbal tea as a caffeine replacement. I recommend chamomile tea or tulsi tea, also known as holy basil. I recommend tulsi tea because it acts as an adaptogen, lowering cortisol levels and improving relaxation.[1]

Another thing that exhausts your organs and causes stressed gut is excessive alcohol consumption. Sure, a glass of wine to start the weekend isn't going to cause problems, but when you drink a couple of glasses two or more times a week, you're triggering an inflammatory reaction in your body. The same goes for beer and hard spirits. Try to restrict yourself to one glass, once a week.

The overconsumption of grains and sugar is one of the most common causes of stressed gut, as they overtax your thyroid and kidneys. Avoiding grains, sugars, breads, and pastas will support your body's attempt to heal itself from stressed gut.

Foods that promote healing contain high levels of vitamin B_{12}, such as grass-fed beef, wild-caught salmon, and fermented dairy like kefir or yogurt. In the past, I've treated a lot of people with stressed gut who were vegans or vegetarians, but I don't believe it's a good idea to embrace either of those restrictive diets if you have stressed gut.

— Your Four-Step Strategy for Healing Stressed Gut —

Stressed gut can be caused by emotional stress that leads to thyroid issues, adrenal fatigue, and elevated cortisol levels. Bacterial imbalance caused by stress can also lead to immune dysfunction, greater risk of infection or sickness, and, if left untreated, eventual autoimmune disease. Review the explanation of stressed gut. What makes sense to you? Do you feel like you're under mental or emotional stress?

1. Eliminate Triggers: Foods Toxic to the Adrenals, Kidneys, and Thyroid

▶ High-sugar foods create swings in blood sugar (a stressor in itself) and mood swings; try to make the connection that "sugar makes me feel worse." Satisfy cravings with fruit or tea.

▶ Grains found in breakfast cereals and "healthy" nutrition bars can quickly turn into sugar and overstress the body. Severely limit any grains (especially highly refined processed grains) in your diet.

▶ Caffeine stimulates the adrenals, can harm the thyroid, and can also put pressure on kidneys and adrenals. Limit yourself to one caffeinated beverage daily.

▶ Alcohol is a depressant that can affect our thoughts, feelings, and actions and provoke anxiety. Drinking is not a positive way to manage stress.

▶ Consuming cold food items, like drinking ice water or constantly eating salads, can make the digestive system work harder than it should. Instead, have a bowl of warm bone broth soup or chicken vegetable soup and drink a warm cup of tea during the day.

2. Consume Therapeutic Foods

▶ Salty foods as well as dark-colored foods—meaning those foods that are purple, black, or blue—are mainstays for those healing stressed gut.

▶ Good salty food options to try are kale chips, miso soup, artichoke hearts, pumpkin seeds, and hummus.

▶ Examples of richly hued foods in purple, black, or blue are blueberries, plums, purple cabbage, eggplant, and purple grapes. Anthocyanins, the phytonutrients responsible for giving purple foods their color, soothe inflammation in the gut.

▶ Foods high in B vitamins, like grass-fed beef, poultry, brewer's yeast, and green leafy vegetables, help regulate mood.

▶ Foods high in calcium, like unsweetened organic yogurt or wild-caught salmon, can reduce anxiety.

▶ Foods high in magnesium, like nuts, avocados, and sea vegetables, calm the nerves. For people deficient in magnesium, these foods can restore balance.

▶ Foods high in protein and amino acids, like bone broth, beef and chicken liver, grass-fed meats from bison and beef, poultry, wild game, and wild-caught fish, support metabolism and hormone balance.

▶ Foods high in omega-3 fatty acids, such as wild cold-water fish, grass-fed meats, and sprouted seeds and nuts, can reduce inflammation and help stabilize mood.

▶ Nutrient-dense foods that are easy to digest and have healing qualities are coconut, olives, avocado, cruciferous vegetables (cauliflower, broccoli, brussels sprouts, etc.), pumpkin seeds, chia seeds, and flaxseeds.

▶ Brazil nuts are a selenium-rich snack that supports the adrenal glands.

▶ Use sea salt—high in electrolytes—instead of the popular iodized salt. Sprinkling a bit of sea salt on meats and vegetables supports hydration.

3. Treat with Supplements

▶ Vitamin B_{12} can restore adrenal function, reduce homocysteine (a toxic amino acid), and increase energy.

▶ Adaptogenic herbs like ashwagandha, rhodiola, tulsi, ginseng, and licorice root extract are nutrients that can help you overcome stressed gut. Ashwagandha improves levels of DHEA, a hormone produced by the adrenal glands, and helps you sleep.

▶ L-glutamine powder is a multipurpose treatment for your stressed gut. This amino acid helps protect, heal, and repair the gut lining while simultaneously reducing stress and depression.

▶ Probiotics can reduce anxiety and are crucial to replenishing the good bacteria needed in the gut, which will support the adrenal glands.

▶ Selenium relieves oxidative stress and supports the thyroid, often compromised in stressed gut.

▶ Fish oil, high in omega-3 fatty acids, will help support adrenal function.

4. Transform Your Lifestyle

▶ Those who experience stressed gut tend to worry, feel anxious, and obsess over life's difficulties. Be serious about reducing the amount of stress in your life. Employ multiple methods, not just one. Aside from reducing sugar and alcohol, this is the core remedy for stressed gut.

▶ To overcome any lingering emotional trauma, support yourself emotionally by becoming part of a faith community or by seeking out good friends you can lean on.

▶ Journal or otherwise release bottled-up emotions that you've been carrying in the pit of your stomach for days, months, or years.

▶ Try to forgive yourself. From my experience with patients, I believe that not forgiving yourself for past actions and carrying feelings of low self-esteem perpetuate stressed gut.

▶ Reduce interactions with people who are negative (and likely cause the stress in our lives!). Write down the names of five people who suck the energy right out of you, who belittle you, or who criticize and second-guess everything you do. Actively think of ways of decreasing contact with these people.

▶ Conversely, write down the names of five people who are the most encouraging, the best listeners, and great supporters. Proactively schedule time to hang out and socialize with these friends, who will help you grow into a better person.

▶ Talk to a therapist, pastor, or trusted friend for counseling. Everyone needs help sometimes and it doesn't reflect on your character to ask for the help you need.

▶ Find three effective stress relievers that work for you. These could be standing up and taking a few deep breaths, stepping outside and walking around the block, running a few errands, or planning something you enjoy doing at the end of your stress-filled day.

▶ Also, find "your thing." Maybe it's a fitness class or a new project associated with your favorite hobby. (My mother loved riding her horse, Jazz, after her school day ended, which helped her tremendously when she was bouncing back from cancer and leaky gut.)

▶ Pay attention to your posture. Stress can physically hobble you to the point where you hunch over. Perk up, straighten your spine, lift your chin, and carry yourself confidently.

▶ Retreat from your get-it-done mind-set and engage in social time to remove yourself from the isolating work vortex. Just like you block out time for your work, you need to schedule "fun time" and "relaxation time" into your weekly planner.

▶ Exercise is one of the best stress busters out there. Give yourself at least thirty minutes every day or every other day for exercise. Having an exercise partner is also great for accountability.

▶ If you love the beach like I do, imagine yourself on the shoreline with the smell of salt air, the squawks of seagulls, and the smell of sunscreen lotion. Soak it all in.

▶ Taking a healing detox bath is one of the best ways to relieve stress. In the evening after dinner, add one cup of Epsom salts and twenty drops of lavender oil to a hot bath and soak for twenty minutes. Then drink a warm glass of chamomile tea.

— Stressed Gut Daily Routine —

7:00 a.m. Upon Waking
Take a few minutes to breathe deeply the moment you get out of bed. Be sure to plan something you can look forward to at the end of your day.

8:00 a.m. Breakfast and Supplements
Enjoy a low-sugar, stressed gut–friendly breakfast. Pack your lunch and snacks (if you didn't the night before) and take your first round of supplements: probiotics, vitamin B, and supplements to support your adrenals and heal from leaky gut.

10 a.m. Morning Break
Drink an eight-to-sixteen-ounce glass of warm herbal tea, like tulsi or licorice tea.

12:00 p.m. Lunch
Lunch can be light with a warm bowl of bone broth soup and a lettuce salad with avocado.

5:00 p.m. Get Active
Make sure you follow through on your after-work plans. Do a fun workout in a group setting like barre, Pilates, or burst training. Or go on a bike ride or a brisk walk through the neighborhood.

6:00 p.m. Dinner and Supplements
Dinner should include foods packed with B vitamins, such as grass-fed beef, and green leafy vegetables, like kale or spinach. Take another round of supplements: probiotics, vitamin B, adrenal support supplements, and adaptogenic herbs, such as ashwagandha and holy basil.

8:00 p.m. Before Bedtime
Time to treat yourself with a nice relaxing bath. Draw hot water and add Epsom salts and twenty drops of lavender oil and soak for twenty minutes.

10:00 or 10:30 p.m. Bedtime
Turn off the TV an hour before bedtime. Resist the temptation to get on social networks. Wind down by reading an uplifting book. Sleep well and get quality rest.

— Stressed Gut Nourishing Foods List —

Meat/Protein (three-to-five-ounce servings)
- kefir (raw, organic)
- yogurt (goat's milk and cultured for twenty-four hours or longer)
- wild-caught fish
- bison
- lean beef
- liver (from chicken or beef)
- turkey
- bone broth
- collagen powder (bone broth in powder form)

Vegetables (cooked)
- asparagus
- broccoli
- brussels sprouts
- carrots
- cauliflower
- chard
- eggplant
- kale
- mushrooms
- sauerkraut
- seaweed
- spinach
- spirulina
- water chestnuts

Fruits (one serving daily maximum)
- avocado
- blackberries
- blueberries
- cranberries
- raspberries
- figs
- pomegranate
- strawberries

Grains (sprouted)
- quinoa
- wild rice

Legumes
- black beans
- kidney beans

Fats/Oils
► avocado
► coconut oil
► ghee (clarified butter)

Flours
► coconut flour

Herbs
► basil
► maca root powder
► sage
► sea salt
► thyme
► turmeric

Sweeteners
► raw honey (maximum of one tablespoon daily)
► stevia

Beverages
► nettle tea
► tulsi teas

Seeds/Nuts (one-tablespoon serving)
► almonds
► black sesame seeds
► Brazil nuts
► chia seeds
► pumpkin seeds
► walnuts

Danger Foods
► alcohol
► caffeinated drinks (including coffee)
► refined grains
► sugar

14

Healing Immune Gut

THE IMMUNE GUT TYPE PRESCRIPTION

Causes	Food sensitivities, gluten, and dairy products.
The Right Diet	Beef bone broth, chicken vegetable soup made from bone stock, and adopting a grain-free diet.
The Right Supplements	Digestive enzymes, probiotics, and L-glutamine.
Good Practices	Listening to your body and knowing that allergic reactions can occur up to forty-eight to seventy-two hours later.

I have good news and bad news for you. The bad news first: the most severe form of leaky gut is immune gut. The good news is that there is hope to heal completely. If you've been diagnosed with autoimmune disease or inflammatory bowel disease like ulcerative colitis, Crohn's disease, or irritable bowel syndrome, then the immune gut healing plan will be a pathway for turning around your troubled and pain-filled life. This diet focuses on reducing immune reactions and giving the body easy-to-digest foods.

Multiple food allergies, sensitivities, and intolerances are some of the biggest warning signs of immune gut. During our lives, most of us will eat more than twenty-five tons of food, and unfortunately, not all of it will be absorbed well by our bodies.[1]

When partially digested protein and fat leaks through your gut lining and into your bloodstream, your body perceives it as a foreign invader and creates an allergic response. You might not start sneezing or break out in a rash. Brain fog, fatigue, and a drop in blood sugar are signs of intolerance, too. It can be hard to identify allergies. In some cases, reactions to allergens don't appear for forty-eight to seventy-two hours.

- ► **Food allergies** are immediate, severe immune responses to IgE antibodies.
- ► **Food sensitivities** are milder, delayed immune responses to IgG antibodies.
- ► **Food intolerances** are metabolic or gastrointestinal responses caused by a lack of enzymes or other inability to digest certain foods.

Whether the response is mild or severe, continuing to eat these foods can lead to serious health issues beyond a leaky gut, such as inflammatory bowel disease, IBS, arthritis, eczema, psoriasis, depression, anxiety, migraine headaches, muscle pain, or chronic fatigue. The best solution we currently have for identifying these allergens is the elimination diet. Although allergy testing can be unreliable (and cannot test for sensitivities and intolerances), an elimination diet has proven to be effective for identifying foods that cause a negative reaction in your gut.

According to ancient Chinese medicine, those experiencing symptoms of immune gut have problems because their primary emotional responses to conflict are insecurity, grief, and a lack of confidence. Those who are detail oriented with perfectionist tendencies are also prime candidates for immune gut because they can't let go of their commitment to do "what's right." In addition, any time a person with immune gut loses a loved one or experiences profound grief, they can experience issues in the gut.

In order to heal yourself of immune gut, you must address these emotions as well as the other precipitating factors that could stem from your intense nature. You will need to become more accepting of change and gracefully release the past. If you don't, you'll put even more stress on your gut.

— The Immune Gut Type Action Plan —

To lessen immune gut's grip, it's critical to avoid the antinutrients that damage your gut lining. I recommend that you keep a food journal, writing down *every* morsel of food that passes your lips. You should also track everything you drink. Keeping a comprehensive log is the best way to understand and control your food sensitivities and/or food allergies while noting any reactions in the body. If your nose is running after that cheese omelet, or you experience joint pains or extreme fatigue after eating a Danish, recording those experiences in a journal will help you turn your life around.

Immune reactions don't necessarily happen right after you finish your last bite of a meal, however. Sometimes adverse reactions crop up twenty-four hours later or even two or three days later. By continually tracking how you're feeling, you can look for patterns that relate to your good days and bad days.

From my clinical experience, I've found that the overuse of prescription antibiotic medications in formative years is a major cause of immune gut. Antibiotics wipe out the good and bad microorganisms in the gut, which over time catches up with you. Eventually, the bad microorganisms rise to levels that leave your gut open to food sensitivities that lead to inflammatory bowel disease.

If you believe you have immune gut from the gut type quiz, the first thing I would recommend that you do is take an IgG (immunoglobulin G) test that checks for food intolerances in the body. If you have a food intolerance issue, there's a strong likelihood you have immune gut.

The IgG test will also give you a list of foods that you're sensitive to, and these are exactly the foods you shouldn't be eating. You must eliminate them from your diet, no matter how difficult that will be. Your long-term health is at stake—and so is your short-term future. Begin your healing by consuming only bone broth, cooked vegetables, and organic chicken. It's also important to eat organically grown vegetables, since those with immune gut often have adverse reactions to the pesticides and herbicides found in conventionally grown produce.

One of the first foods I want you to start incorporating into your diet is bone broth. Whenever somebody asks me, "What's the ideal meal for immune gut?" my answer will always be rich bone broth.

Bone broth can be made from beef bones or chicken parts. For the latter, I like going to a local farmer's market and buying chicken necks, backs, and feet—yes, two weblike feet—and putting them in a slow cooker for twenty-four hours, letting them simmer in water and apple cider vinegar. I'll also add garlic and two onions. This stock is the foundation of a fantastic chicken soup.

Beef bone broth is certainly a great choice as well. You can order beef bones online and have them shipped to your home or go to Whole Foods or a natural food grocer to buy a bag of organic, free-range beef bones. If you're pressed for time, you can purchase already prepared beef bone broth or chicken bone broth online from stores such as Wise Choice Market and U.S. Wellness Meats.

Consume at least one helping a day of bone broth. You can add vegetables like butternut squash, spaghetti squash, or acorn squash to give the broth a heartier taste.

I want you to feel a sense of urgency about this—if the vicious cycle continues, your body will produce immune responses that lead to more serious autoimmune diseases. But if you follow the immune gut plan, I'm confident that you'll see quick results overcoming immune issues.

— The Four-Step Strategy for Healing Immune Gut —

With immune gut, you're dealing with inflammation of the gut, which is immediately followed by an immune or autoimmune reaction. Food sensitivities—usually gluten and dairy—are the reasons behind immune gut. The root causes often stem from a history of taking prescription antibiotics, birth control pills, steroids, or corticosteroids, which are known for wiping out the good bacteria in the gut. You should take an IgG test to determine if you have food sensitivities or food allergies and see a gastrointestinal specialist who can look for inflammatory bowel disease.

1. Eliminate Triggers: Foods That Cause Intestinal Inflammation

▸ Try an "elimination diet" to identify potential food sensitivities and discover what foods might be triggering immune gut symptoms. Start by eliminating the ten most common food allergens, which are:

- milk (because of the A1 casein and lactose)
- egg whites
- wheat
- grains (especially those that contain gluten)
- soy
- shellfish
- peanuts
- tree nuts such as almonds, Brazil nuts, cashews, chestnuts, hazelnuts, pecans, pistachios, and walnuts
- sugar, especially white refined sugar
- alcohol

- Eliminate the entire list for at least four weeks. Reintroduce one food at a time for three days.
- Keep a log of how you feel for up to two days after a food is added.
- Follow the same steps for each food. (If a food causes a reaction—brain fog, light-headedness, itchy skin, etc.— eliminate it. Then wait to introduce the next new food for two days.)
- Sugary treats like muffins, doughnuts, cakes, and cupcakes, and even breakfast cereals or energy bars, are double trouble because of their refined white flour (gluten) and copious sugar. Sugar is highly inflammatory and should be avoided at all costs.
- Alcohol reacts like sugar in the system, causing inflammation. Alcohol is also a depressant that can affect your thoughts, feelings, and actions and provoke anxiety. Steer clear.
- Consuming cold foods—like drinking ice water or constantly eating salads—can make the digestive system work harder than it should. Instead, aim for a bowl of warm bone broth soup or chicken vegetable soup and drink a warm cup of tea during the day.

2. Consume Therapeutic Foods

▶ Meal planning can be a big help because making bone broth—a big part of the immune gut diet—takes foresight and at least one day in a slow cooker. Take a day over the weekend to shop for the ingredients, so you'll have everything on hand.

▶ Start the day with a probiotic smoothie made with gut-friendly goat's milk kefir and sprouted flaxseeds that will give your "good guy" gut bacteria a real boost. (Note: some people with immune gut may need a gentle start with probiotics, to avoid a histamine overreaction. To be safe, start with a half teaspoon of any probiotic food and work up gradually from there.)

▶ Easily digested cooked vegetables include squash of all types, broccoli, cabbage, cauliflower, asparagus, carrots, celery, chard, spinach, kale, and onions.

▶ Foods high in protein and amino acids are very helpful. They include bone broth, beef and chicken liver, grass-fed meats from bison and beef, poultry, wild game, and wild-caught fish. Grilled honey-glazed wild-caught salmon served on a bed of butter lettuce or arugula would be an ideal meal for those with immune gut.

▶ Foods high in omega-3 fatty acids such as wild-caught cold-water fish, grass-fed meats, and sprouted seeds and nuts can reduce inflammation in the gut.

▶ Healthy fats are olive oil, coconut oil, ghee (clarified butter), and flaxseed oil.

3. Treat with Supplements

▶ L-glutamine helps protect, heal, and repair leaky gut and supports the immune system.

▶ Digestive enzymes will help your gut properly break down foods, helping mitigate poor digestion often linked to food allergies.

▶ Probiotics are crucial to replenishing the good bacteria needed in the gut, but stick to SBOs, especially helpful to immune gut types, as many standard probiotics are started in a dairy base. Start with a small dose of SBO probiotic, and work up gradually.

4. Transform Your Lifestyle

▶ To effectively beat immune gut, you must consciously value the act of building joy in your life. People who struggle with immune gut tend to be perfectionists who are self-disciplined, organized, conscientious, and independent. If that sounds like you, give yourself permission to relax enough to allow joy to come back in your life. Build in restorative time, turning down your get-it-done mind-set, and schedule "fun time" into your weekly planner. Make time to spend with loved ones and have fun.

▶ If you're going through one of life's low points or are experiencing a deep loss, pay close attention to how your body responds to different foods. Those experiencing grief or trauma are in a proinflammatory state and are more susceptible to developing leaky gut and immune gut.

▶ I encourage you to develop an "attitude of gratitude" from the moment you get out of bed in the morning until you retire in the evening. One way we can teach ourselves to be grateful is by saying—out loud—what you're grateful for at the start of the day. It may take work to do this, especially at the beginning, but give yourself a chance to bounce back.

▶ Write about your gratitude in a journal: What are you thankful for in your personal life? What do you appreciate about your job? To whom are you indebted for taking you under his or her wing at a key moment in your life?

▶ Leave room for heartache, too. If there are some parts of your life that have been tough or unpleasant, it's okay to give voice to them as well. Sometimes acknowledging out loud, to yourself, that life hasn't gone as you wished—that you're angry, sad, or frustrated to have faced your current challenges—can help you feel grateful for what you *do* have.

▶ Get physically active, especially if you've been on the sidelines because of your immune gut issues. What are your favorite fitness activities? You don't have to start training for a triathlon, but what about taking a half-hour walk? If you've been meaning to commit to a fitness gym or workout program, now is the time to do so—but start slowly and gently, so as not to provoke injury or inflammation.

▸ Dancing is a way to get moving without putting too much strain on your joints. What people like about dancing is the joy of making and completing choreographed steps. Give yourself that great pleasure.

▸ Watch a funny movie on streaming video or DVD. Listening to music can also help you keep stress at bay. Listen to mellow music during your commute instead of the blood pressure–raising news channels.

— Immune Gut Daily Routine —

7:00 a.m. Upon Waking
Take a few minutes to breathe deeply the moment you get out of bed. I believe it's important to start off the day with quiet time, by reading Scripture or inspirational thoughts.

8:00 a.m. Breakfast and Supplements
Enjoy an immune gut–friendly breakfast such as a warm pear smoothie with collagen powder, which is essentially bone broth in powder form. Be sure to log what you eat. Take your first round of supplements: digestive enzymes, SBO probiotics, and a leaky gut support formula with L-glutamine.

12:00 p.m. Lunch
Eat a warm bowl of chicken vegetable bone broth soup. Remember to write down exactly what you eat and how your body feels afterward.

5:00 p.m. Get Active
Do a fun workout in a group setting like barre, Pilates, or burst training. Or go on a bike ride or a brisk walk through the neighborhood.

6:00 p.m. Dinner and Supplements

Be sure your dinner includes servings of warm vegetables and grass-fed beef or pasture-raised chicken. Take another round of supplements: digestive enzymes, SBO probiotics, and a leaky gut support formula with L-glutamine.

8:00 p.m. Before Bedtime

Time to treat yourself with a nice relaxing bath. Draw hot water and add Epsom salts and twenty drops of lavender oil and soak for twenty minutes. Then listen to expressive but soothing music while you wind down. Review what you ate and how you're feeling, looking for any correlations between what you ate and how you felt afterward.

10:00 or 10:30 p.m. Bedtime

Turn off the TV an hour before bedtime. Resist the temptation to get on social networks. Wind down by reading an uplifting book or journaling.
Sleep well and get quality rest.

— Immune Gut Nourishing Foods List —

Meat/Protein (three-to-five-ounce servings)

- bison
- bone broth
- collagen powder (bone broth in powder form)
- chicken
- duck
- egg yolks
- kefir (raw, organic)
- lamb
- lean beef
- turkey
- wild-caught fish
- yogurt (goat's milk and cultured for twenty-four hours or longer)

Vegetables (cooked)

- acorn squash
- asparagus
- broccoli
- butternut squash
- carrots
- cauliflower
- celery
- chard

- cucumber (peeled)
- garlic
- kale
- onions
- pumpkin
- sauerkraut
- spaghetti squash
- squash
- zucchini

Fruits (one serving daily maximum)
- apples (cooked)
- avocado
- blueberries
- cherries
- lemon
- lime
- mango
- pears

Grains (sprouted)
- none when you have immune gut

Legumes
- none when you have immune gut

Fats/Oils
- avocado
- coconut oil
- flaxseed oil
- ghee (clarified butter)
- olive oil

Flours
- coconut flour

Herbs
- fennel
- ginger
- licorice
- mint
- turmeric

Sweeteners
- raw honey (maximum of one tablespoon daily)
- stevia

Beverages
- chamomile tea
- fennel tea
- ginger tea
- marshmallow tea
- mint tea
- warm water with lemon

Seeds/Nuts (one-tablespoon serving)
- chia seeds (sprouted)
- flaxseeds (sprouted)

Danger Foods
- alcohol
- dairy
- raw foods
- refined foods
- packaged foods

15

Healing Gastric Gut

THE GASTRIC GUT TYPE PRESCRIPTION

Causes	Underchewing, overeating, and a slow digestive system.
The Right Diet	Lots of fruits and vegetables, including fermented vegetables, and smaller meals.
The Right Supplements	HCL with pepsin, manuka honey, apple cider vinegar, and digestive enzymes.
Good Practices	Get out of your comfort zone and try fermented vegetables like sauerkraut, kimchi, and miso.

You've just finished eating an excellent meal at a fine restaurant. *And a healthy one!* you tell yourself. All the ingredients, from the grass-fed rib-eye steak to the quinoa, arugula, and avocado salad, were organic.

And yet within an hour of the meal, your bloated stomach feels like it has risen into your chest, leaving you with a burning sensation. What's happening is another round of acid reflux, a severe form of indigestion that occurs when sour- or bitter-tasting fluids flow up into the back of the throat or mouth after eating.

When acid reflux becomes chronic, it turns into gastroesophageal reflux disease, or GERD. The physiological description goes like this:

during the act of swallowing, the muscle at the bottom of the esophagus weakens, allowing food and acid to rise up into the mouth. Left
untreated, GERD can lead to painful bleeding in the esophagus and
increase the risk of developing cancer of the esophagus.

Jonathan V. Wright, MD, author of *Why Stomach Acid Is Good for
You*, claims that half of the American population over fifty years of
age lacks the appropriate amount of stomach acid to fully digest their
food. If this seems odd to you because of all the advertisements for
acid-blocking medications like Nexium, Pepcid, Prevacid, Prilosec, and
Zantac, it's because the American public has been told for years that *too
much* acid is the culprit for gastrointestinal issues like acid reflux and
GERD—when it's exactly the opposite.

Acid reflux and GERD are vivid and unmistakable signs that you
have gastric gut. Bloating, intestinal gas, and excessive bacteria in
the small intestine (known as SIBO, or small intestinal bacteria overgrowth), are also signs of gastric gut. SIBO, when left untreated, can
lead to potentially serious health complications and nutrient deficiencies, including vitamin B_{12}, which can lead to permanent nerve damage.

The main causes of gastric gut, which is a serious condition, are:

▶ a slow digestive system with low levels of stomach acid
▶ antacid use
▶ poor chewing habits
▶ overeating
▶ heightened emotional responses

Any or all of these causes lead to impaired stomach, spleen, and
pancreas function. Overworking and overexertion are the biggest reasons why people come down with gastric gut. Are you consumed by
your job and putting in a lot of overtime? Trying to get a start-up business going? Scrambling to keep the doors open? If so, the pressures
you're feeling place you in danger of having gastric gut.

With gastric gut, your digestive system tends to work more slowly,
meaning food sits in your stomach longer. Over time, pressure rises in
the stomach, causing an *H. pylori* infection. These bacteria can cause
sores, better known as ulcers, in the lining of your stomach or the
upper part of your small intestine.

In a healthy digestive system, the small intestine has relatively low levels of bacteria; the highest concentrations are in the colon. When bad bacteria invade the small intestine, however, SIBO can occur, causing poor nutrient absorption that results in gastric gut. Cardiovascular problems like heart disease and high blood pressure can arise, but stomach issues like acid reflux and GERD are the most notable manifestations.

Addressing your lifestyle and your high-strung emotions is absolutely essential with gastric gut. According to Chinese medicine, those with gastric gut are related to the fire and earth elements and tend to have fiery personalities. If you're the type who's emotionally involved with life, who reacts in passionate ways, then you're a prime candidate for developing gastric gut. Anything you can do to reduce stress and build peace in your life will lessen symptoms. One of the best ways to feel calm is to write in a journal or read inspirational material upon waking and falling asleep.

From a dietary point of view, chewing your food well will help you tremendously, because half-chewed or barely chewed bites of food put stress on the stomach. Don't wolf down your sandwich or salad. Concentrate on chewing in a relaxed manner—thirty chews with each bite of food—so that the enzymes in your saliva can begin breaking down the food. When you chew well, food tastes better, because a dry tongue can't tell how good food tastes.

During the time it takes you to chew your food a couple of dozen times before swallowing, the stomach is producing hydrochloric acid in preparation for breaking down the food once it enters the stomach. The pancreas is also put on notice to start producing enzymes to break down food.

The spleen also has a major role to play during digestion. In ancient Chinese medicine, the spleen is responsible for transforming food into energy the body can use and helps in repairing the lining of the small intestine, but if leaky gut is overtaxing, then the spleen must work extra hard to repair the lining of the small intestine. As for the pancreas, this organ won't be able to produce enzymes when leaky gut is present, sometimes due to chronic fatigue, chronic illness, improper diet, environmental factors, emotional disturbances, and even aging.

Eating too much is another way to develop gastric gut. Overeating expands the stomach and doesn't allow food to pass through in a timely fashion. In order to keep food moving through, your stomach produces additional hydrochloric acid, while the pancreas produces more enzymes—almost to the point where your insulin receptor sites get burned out, a sign of impending diabetes.

Eat until you feel about 70 or 80 percent full, and then put down your fork. If you think you have gastric gut, I'd like you to start eating smaller, more frequent meals. Consider following a 9 a.m., noon, 3 p.m., and 6 p.m. eating schedule. Drink vegetable juice in the morning and consume bone broth at noontime or later in the day. Intermittent fasting—meaning consuming all your meals during a four-to-six-hour window—can also be very beneficial.

Bitter foods are excellent because they help the pancreas produce more enzymes. Kale, broccoli, cauliflower, brussels sprouts, beets, radishes, and arugula are examples of bitter-tasting vegetables; lemons, limes, grapefruit, and olives are examples of tart-tasting fruit; and chamomile, mint, and dandelion are bitter herbs. All help support the gastric gut.

Mineral water is the beverage of choice if you have gastric gut. Even better is adding a tablespoon of apple cider vinegar, bitter herb drops, or citrus peel essential oil to a glass of sparkling mineral water like San Pellegrino. Don't drink sparkling water or any type of liquid during your meals, however. It's better to drink a little bit of water before you eat and throughout the rest of the day.

— The Gastric Gut Type Action Plan —

A few ground rules for treating gastric gut:

Start with eating every three hours or so with smaller portions. Consuming fermented vegetables frequently would be a great idea. Be sure not to eat past 7 p.m. Better yet, eat these three meals between noon and 6 p.m.

Sip a glass of warm water with one tablespoon of apple cider vinegar before eating. Because vinegar is naturally acidic, it will lower the pH in your stomach. If you're drinking caffeine, gradually reduce your intake. You should only drink fluids between meals. When you sit down before your plate of food, remind yourself to chew each bite of food thoroughly.

Plan out your meals for the week so that you're eating as you should for someone with gastric gut. That means making a short grocery list and shopping for the items you need to have on hand for breakfast, lunch, dinner, and snacks.

Start your day with a smoothie, made with gut-friendly goat's milk and sprouted flaxseeds, to boost the amounts of "good guy" gut bacteria. Lunch can be a simple bowl of bone broth, which is incredibly healthy for you. For dinner, consider making my hearty Slow-Cooker Beef and Root Veggie Stew (see page 255). Since it's a slow-cooker recipe, it's easy to make extra for leftovers. Having another meal ready to go is another stress reducer when it comes to planning out meals.

— Your Four-Step Strategy for Healing Gastric Gut —

The main causes of gastric gut are low stomach acid, use of over-the-counter antacid medications, poor chewing, and overeating, which stress the stomach, spleen, and pancreas. Are you living under emotional stress? Focus your efforts on what you can control, namely chewing habits, eating too much, and using antacids. Being overweight and lack of exercise are major causes of gastric gut; make sure to exercise several times a week. On the days you don't work out, take at least a thirty-minute walk. Feelings of anxiety and fear or pushing yourself to your physical limits leaves you vulnerable to gastric gut as well.

1. Eliminate Triggers: Foods Toxic to the Stomach, Spleen, and Pancreas

▸ Fried foods and too many processed oils are hard to digest and can either speed up or slow down digestion, leading to diarrhea or constipation as well as bloating, gas, and digestive discomfort. The worst processed oils are canola, soybean, and cottonseed oil.

- Gluten-containing grains are high in phytic acid, which is difficult for the body to digest. Gluten often causes inflammation of the gut and worsens symptoms of gastric gut.
- Spicy foods containing sriracha sauce or hot peppers can worsen gastric gut symptoms, leading to diarrhea and loose stools.
- Conventional dairy products are missing enzymes, so they make your pancreas work harder to digest them. Conventional dairy also contains hormones, antibiotics, and medications, all of which can hurt your gut.
- Avoid acidic foods such as citrus, tomatoes, cheese, dark chocolate, and alcohol.

2. Consume Therapeutic Foods

- Fresh organic vegetables and fruits are rich in enzymes and antioxidants and easy to digest. Vegetables and fruits, both cooked and raw, should be the foundation of the gastric gut diet.
- Bitter vegetables and herbs—including romaine lettuce, kale, arugula, radishes, dandelion, watercress, collard greens, citrus peel, plums, raspberries, strawberries, rhubarb, parsley, ginger, and turmeric—are helpful foods for dealing with gastric gut.
- Root vegetables—sweet potatoes, carrots, beets, onions, ginger, and garlic—settle well in the stomach.
- Organic meat from grass-fed beef, pasture-raised chicken, venison, duck, turkey, and wild game soothes gastric gut. Fish caught in the wild is a superior source of protein as well.
- Bone broth made from beef bones or chicken carcasses is greatly beneficial.
- Organic kefir and yogurt are the top-two dairy performers, promoting healthy bacteria and soothing the stomach.
- Cabbage juice and sauerkraut balance gastric acid levels.
- Limit water intake during meals to prevent watering down stomach acid.
- Don't eat while stressed, and avoid high-fiber foods.

3. Treat with Supplements

▶ Digestive enzymes ensure thorough digestion by breaking down food particles. Take one to two capsules with the first bite of each meal.

▶ HCL with pepsin (betaine hydrochloric acid with pepsin, an acid that breaks down proteins in the stomach) should be taken with meals that contain meat. Start off with one capsule, working your way up by one capsule per meal until you get a warming sensation in your stomach. When that happens, back down the dosage by one capsule. If you're not eating meat in your meal, don't take this supplement. Otherwise, you will have an upset stomach.

▶ A word of caution about HCL with pepsin: do not take HCL supplements if you're taking corticosteroids or anti-inflammatory medications like Advil or Tylenol. These drugs could damage the gastrointestinal lining and put you at risk of developing stomach ulcers.

▶ Manuka honey has antimicrobial properties and destroys *H. pylori* bacteria in the stomach. Enjoy one to three teaspoons daily.

▶ Apple cider vinegar promotes the increase of digestive enzymes. Add a tablespoon of apple cider vinegar to a glass of water before meals.

▶ Take a leaky gut support supplement containing L-glutamine, ginger, licorice root, and slippery elm.

▶ Live probiotics that contain soil-based organisms (SBOs) help balance out intestinal flora while improving digestion.

4. Transform Your Lifestyle

▶ According to ancient Chinese medicine, those who experience gastric gut tend to have digestive issues because their primary emotional responses to conflict are being overdramatic and/or aggressive.

▶ Those with gastric gut are social creatures inclined to have fun, likable, and exciting personalities. The difficulties come when emotions run high with their relationships—emotions that work well when things are going as expected but can splinter when things turn negative. In order to completely heal from gastric gut, you must address the emotions in your life and look at your life with logic and a clear mind.

▸ If you have a fiery disposition and are passionate about life and people, your chief emotions are happiness and joy. On the flip side, if you experience the loss of love or great disappointment in a relationship, your chief emotions are frustration, jealousy, regret, and grief.

▸ Those who are wired emotionally as empathetic "heart people" can hurt their stomach, pancreas, spleen, and small intestine function when people let them down or when sad moments occur. Life's disappointments often prompt digestive issues that include leaky gut.

▸ Laughter is one of the most powerful forms of medicine in the world. Schedule times to hang out with friends who make you laugh and lift you up. Fun, easy friendships can be a wonderful tonic.

▸ Look for someone to praise, and let them know you appreciate their work. Sometimes it's easy to focus on ourselves and our issues, but when you look around and see who needs encouragement, lifting their spirits will lift yours as well. Looking for good qualities in others and vocally praising them will give you joy.

▸ Try tai chi, barre, yoga, or some other form of relaxing exercise to calm you.

▸ Treat yourself to a full-body massage, which will do wonders to soothe your mind and body.

— Gastric Gut Daily Routine —

7:00 a.m. Upon Waking

Upon waking, take a few minutes to go over everything that you're grateful for. Then spend five minutes reading an encouraging or inspirational book.

8:00 a.m. Breakfast and Supplements

Before breakfast, sip a glass of water with a tablespoon of apple cider vinegar. Then have a kefir and flaxseed smoothie or light breakfast. Pack your lunch and snacks (if you didn't the night before) and take your first round of supplements: digestive enzymes and any other choice supplements.

12:00 p.m. Lunch

Lunch can be light with a warm bowl of bone broth soup and a lettuce salad with avocado. Take your time while eating and be sure to chew your food thoroughly. Take one or two digestive enzymes and any other choice supplements.

5:00 p.m. Get Active

Do a fun workout in a group setting like barre, Pilates, or burst training. Or go on a bike ride or take a brisk walk through the neighborhood.

6:00 p.m. Dinner and Supplements

Before dinner, sip a glass of water with a tablespoon of apple cider vinegar. Enjoy a light but filling evening meal from the recommend foods list with a healthy snack or dessert afterward. Remind yourself to chew slowly—about thirty times per mouthful. Savor the flavors. Take one or two digestive enzymes and any other choice supplements.

8:00 p.m. Before Bedtime

Time to go into relax mode. Treat yourself with a nice healing bath. Draw hot water and add Epsom salts and twenty drops of lavender oil and soak for twenty minutes. Then relax with your favorite TV show or movie.

10:00 or 10:30 p.m. Bedtime

Turn off the TV an hour before bedtime. Resist the temptation to get on social networks. Wind down by reading an uplifting book. Meditate for a few minutes so you can turn your mind off. Sleep well and get quality rest. When you sleep well, your body produces melatonin and prolactin, a pair of hormones that improve the good bacteria in our gut.

— Gastric Gut Nourishing Foods List —

Meat/Protein (three-to-five-ounce servings)

▶ bison
▶ bone broth
▶ collagen powder
▶ chicken
▶ kefir (raw, organic)
▶ liver (chicken or beef)
▶ lean beef

▶ protein powder (organic)
▶ turkey
▶ wild-caught fish
▶ wild game
▶ yogurt (goat's milk and cultured for twenty-four hours or longer)

Vegetables

▶ arugula
▶ asparagus
▶ beets
▶ bok choy
▶ cabbage
▶ carrots
▶ celery
▶ collard greens
▶ kale
▶ kimchi

▶ pickles
▶ radishes
▶ romaine lettuce
▶ rutabaga
▶ sauerkraut
▶ spaghetti squash
▶ spinach
▶ squash
▶ sweet potatoes
▶ watercress

Fruits

▶ apples
▶ kiwi
▶ mango

▶ papaya
▶ pears
▶ pineapple

Grains (sprouted)

▶ jasmine rice

Legumes

▶ chickpeas (hummus)
▶ mung beans

▶ peas

Fats/Oils

- coconut oil
- flaxseed oil
- ghee (clarified butter)
- olive oil

Flours

- coconut flour

Herbs

- aloe vera
- dill
- fennel
- ginger
- parsley
- peppermint
- turmeric

Sweeteners

- manuka honey (maximum of one tablespoon daily)
- molasses
- stevia

Beverages

- apple cider vinegar
- mineral water (like San Pellegrino)

Seeds/Nuts (one-tablespoon serving)

- chia seeds
- flaxseeds
- hemp seeds
- pumpkin seeds

Danger Foods

- alcohol
- caffeine
- fried foods
- peppers

16

Healing Toxic Gut

THE TOXIC GUT TYPE PRESCRIPTION

Causes	Overconsumption of bad fats and toxicity from the environment, personal care products, and processed foods impair the liver and gallbladder.
The Right Diet	Organically raised meat and fish and organic vegetables and fruits.
The Right Supplements	Probiotics, digestive enzymes with lipase, ox bile, and liver-supportive herbs like milk thistle.
Good Practices	Sour foods and the more raw vegetables, the better!

When any of your organs are not working right, the rest of your body works harder to take up the slack. The high-fat/low-fiber diet of our culture is especially hard on our liver and gallbladder, which help digest fatty foods. An estimated twenty million Americans have gallbladder disease.[1]

The liver, the second-largest organ of the body, filters out harmful oils and toxins in the bloodstream and produces an important digestive liquid known as bile that digests fats and breaks down hormones. The liver also stores essential vitamins and minerals, including iron. When the liver is overloaded and backed up, however, the organ cannot function optimally, which also affects its "paired" organ, the gallbladder. The gallbladder, a small pear-shaped pouch tucked behind the lobes of the liver, stores cholesterol-rich bile that's been secreted by the liver.

Seventy percent of all cases of gallstones form as a result of the body's bile becoming supersaturated with cholesterol. A slow-moving intestinal tract and constipation can also contribute to gallstones. Gallbladder and liver problems can be caused by obesity, rapid weight loss, oral contraceptives, constipation, high-fat diets, high-sugar diets, low-fiber diets, food allergies, and heredity.

When your liver is taxed by the overconsumption of hydrogenated fats and toxins in foods, bile isn't secreted at the correct levels, which places more stress on the small intestine to break down the fats and toxins. When this occurs, your small intestine gets overwhelmed and areas along the intestinal wall open up the tight junctions, allowing the harmful fats and toxins into the bloodstream. This causes inflammation in the digestive tract as well as toxic gut, which ultimately leads to leaky gut. If these symptoms continue over time, the result is malabsorption of fatty acids, gallbladder disease, and often skin inflammation issues like rosacea or neurological diseases.

Traditional Chinese medicine states that the liver and gallbladder can be greatly affected by the emotions of anger, frustration, and a lack of forgiveness. If you're impatient or get frequently frustrated, those emotions directly affect the liver and gallbladder. As a toxic gut type myself, I know forgiving others is hard, especially if you've been wronged. But even if you've dealt with traumatic experiences in life, you must take the first step to forgive anyway.

If you have toxic gut, I recommend that you get a sheet of paper and write down all the people you need to forgive as part of a healing exercise. Then send that person a note or an email saying, "Hey, I just want you to know that I've forgiven you for what's happened between us in the past. I wish you the best." Even better than a handwritten note would be to deliver the message in person. If that's not possible (or advisable), meet with a close friend and tell him or her what happened and why you're forgiving the person who offended you.

Sometime during this process, you may need to meet with a counselor. I can assure you that it's worth the money. One of the best books on the topic of forgiveness is *Do Yourself a Favor . . . Forgive,* by Joyce Meyer, who shows you how to break free of negative thought patterns, control your feelings, and properly deal with frustrations in your life.

Relieving frustration will reduce the stress you feel. Sometimes relief comes from something as simple as getting outside and taking in the beauty of the outdoors. Decluttering and cleaning up around the house will feel like a heavy sack has been lifted from your shoulders. Giving yourself time to meet a best friend for lunch, walk around the mall, or play a recreational sport like tennis or golf can be relaxing.

If you're been going, going, going, then jump off the merry-go-round of life and give your liver and gallbladder a chance to heal from toxic gut.

— The Toxic Gut Type Action Plan —

Turning toxic gut around starts with making changes in the foods you eat so that you can support the liver and gallbladder. Chinese medicine teaches us that those with toxic gut tend to be the wood element, meaning the season of the year they relate to best is springtime. Springtime is when grasses grow, flowers come out, and trees bud—and the world turns green. Thus, the best foods for those with toxic gut will be green:

- ▶ green vegetables like artichokes, broccoli, brussels sprouts, collard greens, sprouts, and watercress
- ▶ green, leafy salads
- ▶ green apples
- ▶ vegetable juices made with carrots, cucumbers, celery, and a shot of wheatgrass

These "live" foods are also full of enzymes, perfect to support your liver and gallbladder. While not green, beets and sour foods like sauerkraut and kimchi are also helpful. For beverages, try dandelion tea or milk thistle tea, as both of these cleanse the liver and gallbladder.

— The Four-Step Strategy for Healing Toxic Gut —

The root causes of toxic gut are stress on the liver and gallbladder as well as not letting go of anger and frustration in your life. You will want to focus your efforts on restoring the health of your liver and gallbladder through diet and learning to forgive and release any frustrations in your personal life. Overeating excess amounts of fatty and chemically laden foods is also hard on the liver and gallbladder, impairing function.

1. Eliminate Triggers: Foods Toxic to the Liver and Gallbladder

- ▶ Fried foods and the hydrogenated and partially hydrogenated oils in processed foods cause a sluggish gallbladder. All high-fat foods, even healthy fats, can cause problems when the gallbladder is weakened, so stay away from nuts, nut butters, lard, and oils.
- ▶ Refined white sugar and simple carbohydrates increase the likelihood of gallstones. Artificial sweeteners are no better, as they're toxic to the liver.
- ▶ Avoid nonorganic foods. Conventionally grown produce and processed foods contain pesticides and GMOs, which are toxic to the liver. Conventionally processed dairy products contain hormones, antibiotics, omega-6 fats, and medications, all of which place tremendous stress on the liver. Pork and conventionally raised meats are high in fats that increase inflammation of the liver.

2. Consume Therapeutic Foods

- ▶ Quality protein sources are antibiotic-free chicken and turkey, grass-fed beef, bison, wild-caught fish, organic protein powder, and real bone broth.
- ▶ Sour foods are the most therapeutic foods for the liver and gallbladder, according to both Chinese and Western medicine. The top sour foods to heal toxic gut are:
  - ▶ asparagus
  - ▶ bok choy
  - ▶ celery

- citrus fruits
- green apples
- kefir
- kimchi
- mung beans
- olives
- plums
- rye sourdough bread
- sauerkraut
- sprouts
- Swiss chard
- yogurt

- Many of the foods in that list are high in fiber. Aim for thirty to forty grams of fiber per day.
- A diet high in raw fruits and vegetables reduces the incidence of gallstones. Consume lots of large salads and vegetable juices.
- Beets, artichokes, and dandelion greens are three vegetables that improve bile flow and break down fats.
- Coconut oil is easier to digest than other fats and oils, but use this fat in moderation.
- Beef and chicken liver are high in nutrients such as vitamin B_{12}, folate, biotin, choline, and vitamin A, which support liver function.
- When you sprout flaxseeds, chia seeds, hemp seeds, and pumpkin seeds, they become more digestible and can reduce inflammation. Eat just one or two tablespoons daily of these sprouted seeds.
- The top beverages are apple cider vinegar mixed in water and chamomile tea.

3. Treat with Supplements

- Digestive enzymes high in lipase improve the digestion of fats and the use of bile. Take one or two capsules daily with meals that contain fat.
- Ox bile/bile salt increases the breakdown of fats. Take five hundred to a thousand milligrams with meals that contain

fat if you aren't digesting fats or have had your gallbladder removed.

▸ Live probiotics with soil-based organisms support detoxification of organs and improve digestion of nutrients and the healing of leaky gut. Take two to four capsules daily.

▸ Liver detox supplements with milk thistle aid the liver in detoxification. Take 150 milligrams twice daily.

▸ Green superfood powder contains wheatgrass juice, chlorella, cilantro, and other cleansing herbs that can improve liver function.

▸ Dandelion, turmeric, and artichoke extract also support the liver in a similar way and can be found in combination formulas.

4. Transform Your Lifestyle

▸ According to traditional Chinese medicine (TCM), those who experience liver and gallbladder issues tend to have those problems because of their "wiring" and their primary emotional responses of anger and frustration when facing conflicts. In order to completely heal toxic gut, you must address toxic emotions as well as attitudes such as unforgiveness and self-righteousness.

▸ In order to reduce the total toxicity of your mind, body, and emotions, begin by making a list of people you haven't forgiven. Then forgive them by speaking their names out loud or by reaching out to those people and letting them know how you were offended but that you've also forgiven them. You may also consider working through forgiveness issues with the help of a counselor.

▸ Practice relaxed, focused thinking or meditation. Take ten to thirty minutes in the morning, around lunch or before bed, and meditate on what you are grateful for and the future you want for yourself.

▸ Go on a daily walk for fifteen to thirty minutes in serene surroundings while deliberately taking cleansing, relaxing breaths of fresh air.

▸ Schedule relaxation time. Often, people with an achievement mentality don't get enough rest, which is toxic to the liver. Take one day a week completely off from work and then schedule fun times during your week.

▶ Getting more sleep is important for those with toxic gut because the body—and especially the liver—cleanses itself while you sleep from 1 a.m. to 3 a.m., according to TCM.

— Toxic Gut Daily Routine —

7:00 a.m. Upon Waking

Upon waking, resist the urge to get on your smartphone or check your email. Instead, take a few minutes to go over everything that you're grateful for. Spend five or ten minutes reading an inspirational book. Focus on being kind, understanding, and gracious in all of your interactions during the day. Then treat yourself to a warm cup of chamomile or dandelion tea.

8:00 a.m. Breakfast and Supplements

Start your day with an organic probiotic-rich yogurt sprinkled with fruit or a green smoothie. Take your first round of supplements: one probiotic capsule, one cell detox capsule, one or two digestive enzymes (if your breakfast contains fats), five hundred milligrams of ox bile/ox bile salt (if your breakfast contains fats), and one scoop of green superfood powder.

12:00 p.m. Lunch and Supplements and After-Lunch Walk

Driven people often work right through lunch, but don't! Instead, consume a healthy lunch, such as a warm bowl of bone broth soup and a lettuce salad with avocado. Take your next round of supplements: one probiotic capsule, one cell detox capsule, one or two digestive enzymes (if your lunch contains fats), and five hundred milligrams of ox bile/ox bile salt (if your lunch contains fats).

2:30 or 3 p.m. Afternoon Snack

Refuel your energy levels or blood sugar levels with a midafternoon snack from toxic gut–friendly foods. You could also have a scoop of green powder with a large glass of water to support energy.

5:00 p.m. Get Active

Do a fun workout in a group setting, such as barre, Pilates, burst training, or weight training, or anything else that is fun, social, and gets your heart rate up.

6:00 p.m. Dinner and Supplements

Find a good place to stop with your work and go home for dinner. Enjoy a light but filling evening meal from the recommended foods list with a healthy snack or dessert afterward. Take your supplements: one probiotic capsule, one cell detox capsule, one or two digestive enzymes (if your dinner contains fats), and five hundred milligrams of ox bile/ox bile salt (if your dinner contains fats). Remind yourself to chew slowly—about thirty times per mouthful. Savor the flavors.

8:00 p.m. Before Bedtime

Have a calming herbal tea, such as chamomile, to wind down. Treat yourself with a soothing bath. Draw hot water and add Epsom salts and twenty drops of lavender oil and soak for twenty minutes. Then relax with your favorite TV show or movie.

10:00 or 10:30 p.m. Bedtime

Turn off the TV an hour before bedtime. Resist the temptation to get on social networks. Wind down by reading an uplifting book. Prioritize sleep, as it keeps you healthy physically, mentally, emotionally, and even spiritually. Deep sleep encourages release of melatonin and prolactin, hormones that support the good bacteria in your gut.

— Toxic Gut Nourishing Foods List —

Meat/Protein (three-to-five-ounce servings)

- bison
- bone broth
- collagen powder
- chicken
- kefir (raw, organic)
- liver (chicken or beef)
- lean beef
- protein powder (organic)
- turkey
- wild-caught fish
- yogurt (goat's milk and cultured for twenty-four hours or longer)

Vegetables

- artichokes
- arugula
- asparagus
- beets
- bell peppers
- bok choy
- carrots
- celery
- cucumber
- kale
- kimchi
- pickles
- radishes
- romaine lettuce
- sauerkraut
- spinach
- spirulina
- sprouts
- vegetable juices (fresh pressed)

Fruits

- blackberries
- blueberries
- grapes (dark)
- grapefruit
- green apples
- lemons
- limes
- plums
- raspberries

Grains (sprouted)

- oats
- rye

Legumes

- green lentils
- lima beans
- mung beans

Fats/Oils
- avocados
- coconut oil
- flaxseed oil

Flours
- coconut flour

Herbs
- cilantro
- citrus peel
- cumin
- dandelion
- garlic
- milk thistle
- turmeric

Sweeteners
- raw honey
- stevia

Beverages
- apple cider vinegar
- dandelion tea
- water with lemon

Seeds/Nuts (one-tablespoon serving)
- black sesame seeds
- chia seeds
- flaxseeds
- hemp seeds
- pumpkin seeds

Danger Foods
- alcohol
- conventional dairy
- fried foods
- nut butters
- oils

part four

THE EAT DIRT RECIPES

17

———

Recipes for Home and Body

W hat better place to get dirty than in the kitchen? As we start to move away from industrial food and cleaning and personal care products, we open ourselves up to an entire world of new flavors, scents, and sensory experiences.

In the first section of this chapter, I've collected many of the essential oil blend recipes I share with my patients who are transitioning away from chemical cleaners and personal care products. Thereafter, I've gathered more than a hundred recipes, from breakfast and smoothies, main dishes, and snacks to side dishes and desserts—everything you need to get started nourishing your body's healthy microbes and healing and sealing your gut lining. If you are just following the Eat Dirt core program from chapter 10, you can choose from any of the recipes in this chapter. If you are following the protocol of one of the five gut types, you can focus on the recipes for that one type, as those dishes have been designed to include many of the healing foods that gut type needs. All of the recipes emphasize foods that tend to be high in soil-based organism probiotics and helpful digestive enzymes, as well as types of prebiotic fiber and high-quality fats that beneficial bacteria and healing guts love most.

As you start to use these recipes, please leave yourself plenty of time in the kitchen to thoroughly enjoy the experience. Plan out a few recipes ahead of time, so you can be sure to have all the ingredients at hand when the time is right. Then, as you crack every egg and chop every onion, as you measure every drop of essential oil, you can revel in how getting dirty is helping your body get healthy. Enjoy!

— The Eat Dirt Home-Care Products —

We'll start with the products you can use around the house to clean and beautify your home. All of these ingredients can be found online, in your local health food store, and sometimes even in a standard grocery store. The homemade tea tree and lemon household cleaner is good for cleaning just about anything in the home—floors, sinks, countertops, and toilets. And since many commercial dishwashing detergents contain a slew of toxic chemicals—and because your family will be better off with more hand-washed dishes and glasses—I suggest that you use a natural brand of dishwashing soap or make your own.

After spending a lifetime thinking that "killing bugs on contact" is the equivalent of clean, you may need some time to get used to the idea that natural products *can* make things clean. But just keep reminding yourself that rather than help your family stay healthy, those harsh chemical cleansers actually put their health at risk. Please know and have faith that your home will be much safer without that kind of anti-microbial warfare.

HOMEMADE HOUSE CLEANER

8 ounces water

4 ounces distilled white vinegar

15 drops tea tree essential oil

15 drops lemon oil

glass spray bottle

1. Add all ingredients to spray bottle.
2. Close bottle and shake to mix.
3. Swirl or shake bottle before you spray.

HOMEMADE DISHWASHING DETERGENT

½ cup liquid castile soap   1 tablespoon white vinegar

2 drops essential oils of your choice   ½ cup water

Combine all ingredients and pour into a BPA-free plastic bottle.

HOMEMADE LAUNDRY SOAP

1 bar of grated castile soap   1 cup baking soda

2 cups borax   15 drops lavender essential oil

2 cups washing soda   15 drops peppermint essential oil

Combine all ingredients and store in an airtight container.

— Eat Dirt Self-Care Products —

Have you started using essential oils yet? I've found that when people make the transition from industrial self-care products to these DIY recipes, they are amazed at not only how fresh and clean they feel, but how the oils can help them focus, feel calmer and happier, and generally get stronger and healthier. They tell me that after the initial transition, they feel much safer knowing that these oils are not destroying their gut. Can you get all of that from a chemical-based hand sanitizer? I don't think so!

HOMEMADE HAND SANITIZER

3 tablespoons aloe vera gel   1 teaspoon vitamin E

1 tablespoon filtered water   squeeze bottle

5 drops tea tree essential oil

1. Combine all ingredients and mix.
2. Transfer ingredients into squeeze bottle.

HOMEMADE PROBIOTIC TOOTHPASTE

¼ cup coconut oil

3 tablespoons bentonite clay

2 capsules of probiotics

10 drops of peppermint essential oil

silicone tube

1. Mix all ingredients together.
2. Put into silicone tube or sealed glass container.
3. Brush teeth for 2 minutes, 2 or 3 times daily.

HOMEMADE LAVENDER SOAP BAR

20–30 drops of lavender essential oil

soap base

3 drops of vitamin E

soap mold of your choice

1. Put soap base in glass bowl and then place bowl in saucepan with water.
2. Heat stove to medium and allow base to melt.
3. Remove from heat and let cool slightly. Then add the lavender and vitamin E.
4. Mix well and transfer to a soap mold.
5. Let mixture cool fully before popping bar out of mold.

HOMEMADE ROSEMARY MINT SHAMPOO

6 ounces aloe vera gel

3 tablespoons olive oil

10 tablespoons baking soda

20 drops rosemary essential oil

10 drops peppermint essential oil

BPA-free plastic dispenser bottle or glass bottle

1. Combine all ingredients in a bowl and mix well.
2. Transfer to a container. Mix well before each use.

HOMEMADE BODY WASH

1 cup water

¼ cup honey

⅔ cup liquid castile soap

30 drops lavender, chamomile, or geranium essential oils

1 teaspoon vitamin E

2 teaspoons jojoba oil

BPA-free plastic lotion dispenser or glass bottle with dispenser

Mix ingredients until smooth and store in 8-ounce bottle.

HOMEMADE FRANKINCENSE AND MYRRH BODY LOTION

¼ cup olive oil

¼ cup coconut oil

¼ cup beeswax

¼ cup shea butter

2 tablespoons vitamin E

20 drops frankincense essential oil

20 drops myrrh essential oil

BPA-free plastic lotion dispenser bottles

1. Put olive oil, coconut oil, beeswax, and shea butter in glass bowl, then place the bowl in saucepan with water.
2. Heat stove to medium and mix ingredients together.
3. Once mixed, put in refrigerator for an hour until solid.
4. With a regular mixer or hand mixer, beat the mixture until it is whipped and fluffy. Then add vitamin E and essential oils and mix.
5. Fill containers and store in cool place.

HOMEMADE MUSCLE RUB

½ cup coconut oil

¼ cup grated beeswax

2 teaspoons cayenne powder

2 teaspoons ginger or turmeric powder

15 drops peppermint essential oil

15 drops lavender essential oil

glass jar

metal tins or storage containers

1. Put coconut oil and beeswax into a jar. Place a saucepan with 2 inches of water over medium-low heat.
2. Place jar in saucepan and allow contents to melt. Stir to combine. Add the cayenne and ginger/turmeric.
3. Once combined, allow to cool slightly and then add essential oils. Mix well.
4. Pour mixture into metal tins or storage containers and allow to set.

HOMEMADE VAPOR RUB

¼ cup olive oil

½ cup coconut oil

¼ cup grated beeswax

20 drops peppermint essential oil

20 drops eucalyptus essential oil

glass jar

metal tins or storage containers

1. Pour olive oil, coconut oil, and beeswax into a jar. Place a saucepan with 2 inches of water over medium-low heat.
2. Place jar in saucepan and allow oils to melt. Stir to combine.
3. Once combined, allow to cool slightly and then add essential oils. Mix well.
4. Pour mixture into metal tins or storage containers and allow to set.

HOMEMADE POMEGRANATE LIP BALM

2 tablespoons beeswax

1 teaspoon coconut oil

1 tablespoon olive oil

1 teaspoon honey

7 drops pomegranate oil

lip balm tins or lip balm tubes

1. In a small pot over medium-low heat, melt beeswax, coconut oil, and olive oil. Use chopstick or other small, long stick to stir.
2. Remove from heat and add honey and pomegranate oil. Whisk well with chopstick and try to distribute oil throughout the mixture.
3. Pour quickly into tins or jars. Let cool on counter till hard.

HOMEMADE SUNBURN SPRAY

½ cup water

⅓ cup aloe vera gel

10 drops lavender essential oil

10 drops frankincense essential oil

5 drops peppermint essential oil

blue glass spray bottle

1. Place all ingredients in a bowl and mix together.
2. Transfer mixture into a spray bottle. Shake well before each use.

HOMEMADE DEODORANT

½ cup coconut oil

½ cup baking soda

40–60 drops essential oils—your choice
of scents

empty deodorant containers

(Recommended scents for women: lavender, ylang-ylang, and sage; recommended scents for men: cedarwood, cypress, clove, rosemary, and bergamot.)

1. Put coconut oil in bowl.
2. Mix in baking soda.
3. Add essential oils.
4. Store in a deodorant container or a glass jar and apply topically to underarms.

HOMEMADE HORMONE BALANCE SERUM

3 ounces evening primrose oil

30 drops clary sage oil

30 drops thyme oil

30 drops ylang-ylang oil

glass vial with dropper

1. Mix all ingredients together.
2. Put into glass vial with dropper.
3. Rub 5 drops onto neck 2 times daily.

HOMEMADE FOCUS AND MEMORY BLEND

5 milliliters cedarwood oil   5 milliliters peppermint oil

5 milliliters vetiver oil   glass vial with dropper

1. Mix all ingredients together.
2. Put into glass vial with dropper.
3. Rub 5 drops onto neck 2 times daily.

If you like these, you can find more home remedies, such as an avocado face mask, bath salts, cellulite cream, hair conditioner, and cough syrup, on my website at DrAxe.com. Let these natural Earth-based remedies help you reach your highest level of health.

— The Eat Dirt Recipes —

What better way to eat dirt than via your fork? These meals are packed with vital nutrients that will help rebalance the microbes in your gut, soothe and seal your gut lining, and ensure healthy, regular digestion to keep the whole system on an even keel. The recipes are organized by gut type, to emphasize those foods and nutrients most critical to that specific type's unique needs. But all of these recipes use the Eat Dirt core principles, and any recipe in this section will help to keep you and your microbiome well fed and happy. Feel free to select any that appeal to you.

Candida Gut Recipes

These recipes are specifically designed to help you eliminate yeast and bacterial overgrowth.

Beverages & Breakfasts

MORNING REFRESHER SMOOTHIE

TOTAL TIME: **5 minutes** | SERVES: **1 or 2**

½ bunch spinach

½ banana

½ cucumber, peeled

½ cup goat's milk kefir

½ cup ice

1 scoop protein powder

1 teaspoon cinnamon

water

In a high-powered blender, combine all ingredients, adding water as necessary. Puree on high until smooth.

COCONUT CREPES

TOTAL TIME: **30 minutes** | SERVES: **4 or 5**

6 eggs

1 cup coconut milk

3 tablespoons coconut flour

3 teaspoons coconut oil, melted, plus additional for greasing pan

½ teaspoon sea salt

1. In a medium bowl, combine all ingredients. Beat with electric mixer for 3 minutes. Let stand 15 minutes.
2. Heat skillet greased with coconut oil over medium-high heat. Ladle batter into pan and swirl around to form a thin crepe. Cook until bubbles start to form, 1–2 minutes. Flip and cook until golden. Repeat with remaining batter.

TURMERIC EGGS

TOTAL TIME: **25 minutes** | SERVES: **2**

3 tablespoons ghee

½ cup chopped onion

8 scallions, chopped

6 cloves garlic, minced

2 tablespoons turmeric

4 eggs

1 tablespoon chopped fresh thyme

1 tablespoon chopped fresh oregano

1 tablespoon chopped fresh basil leaves

(continued on next page)

1. In a medium skillet over medium-low heat, melt ghee. Add onion, scallions, garlic, and turmeric. Cook until vegetables are softened, about 10 minutes.

2. In a medium bowl, combine eggs and herbs. Add to skillet and cook, stirring constantly, until desired doneness.

Soups & Salads

CURRIED CAULIFLOWER SOUP

TOTAL TIME: 40 minutes | SERVES: 4

1 onion, chopped

1 cauliflower head, cut into florets

2 tablespoons coconut oil

1 teaspoon sea salt, plus a pinch

1 teaspoon pepper

3 cups chicken bone broth

½ teaspoon coriander

½ teaspoon turmeric

1½ teaspoons cumin

1 pound chicken, cooked and shredded

1 cup coconut milk

2 tablespoons chopped parsley

1. Preheat oven to 375 degrees F. Spread out onion and cauliflower on a baking sheet. Drizzle with the coconut oil and season with 1 teaspoon each of the sea salt and pepper. Roast for 10 minutes. Stir and place back in the oven for another 5–10 minutes, until golden.

2. Place the cauliflower and onions in a pot and add the bone broth. Stir in the coriander, turmeric, cumin, and a pinch of sea salt. Bring mixture to a boil. Reduce the heat to medium and let mixture simmer for another 5–10 minutes.

3. Add the heated mixture to a high-powered blender and puree until a smooth consistency is achieved. Return to the pot and add the chicken, coconut milk, and parsley. Mix until well combined and serve warm.

SLOW-COOKER LEMON-KALE CHICKEN SOUP

TOTAL TIME: 6½ hours | SERVES: 6–8

2 pounds boneless, skinless chicken
   breasts, chopped

6 cups chicken bone broth

1 onion, chopped

3 handfuls chopped kale

½ cup fresh lemon juice

sea salt and pepper

2 tablespoons chopped fresh parsley

1. In a slow cooker, combine chicken, broth, onion, kale, and lemon juice. Season with salt and pepper.
2. Cook on low for 6–8 hours. Stir in parsley. Taste and adjust seasoning if necessary.

CHICKEN BONE BROTH

TOTAL TIME: 24 hours | SERVES: Varies

2 to 3 chicken necks and feet
  (or carcass of roast chicken)
garlic cloves, smashed
carrots, cut into chunks
onions, cut into chunks

spinach
3 tablespoons apple cider vinegar
2 bay leaves
sea salt and pepper
water

1. In a slow cooker, combine all ingredients with enough water to completely cover chicken parts.
2. Cook on high and allow to simmer for 24 hours.
3. Strain, cool, transfer to airtight storage containers, and chill or freeze.

Main Dishes

SLOW-COOKER BEEF AND ROOT VEGGIE STEW

TOTAL TIME: 4½ hours | SERVES: 4–6

2 pounds cubed grass-fed beef stew
  meat
2 sweet potatoes, peeled and diced
2 onions, chopped
1 rutabaga, peeled and diced
4 carrots, chopped

2 cloves garlic, minced
2 cups beef bone broth
2 tablespoons Worcestershire sauce
1 teaspoon apple cider vinegar
sea salt and pepper

1. In a slow cooker, combine all ingredients and mix well.
2. Cook on high for 4–6 hours. Season to taste.

AVOCADO-STUFFED MEATBALLS

TOTAL TIME: **30 minutes** | SERVES: **4**

coconut oil (for greasing pan)

1 pound ground grass-fed beef

1 egg

3 tablespoons chopped fresh parsley

4 cloves garlic, minced

1 tablespoon Dijon mustard

1 teaspoon sea salt

1 teaspoon pepper

½ avocado, cut into small dice

1. Preheat oven to 400 degrees F. Lightly grease sheet pan with coconut oil.
2. In large bowl, combine all remaining ingredients except avocado. Mix well and, using wet hands, form 8 to 12 meatballs.
3. To stuff meatballs, make a hole in center, insert avocado cube, and close up hole, making sure avocado is fully surrounded by meat.
4. Place meatballs on prepared sheet pan and bake until cooked through, about 12 minutes.

SAUSAGE AND SAUERKRAUT

TOTAL TIME: **30 minutes** | SERVES: **4**

2 tablespoons coconut oil, melted

4 rutabagas, peeled and cubed

1 onion, sliced

1 pound organic chicken sausage, cut
    into ¼-inch pieces

16 ounces sauerkraut, drained

¼ teaspoon pepper

½ teaspoon sea salt

1. In a large skillet, sauté the rutabaga in the coconut oil for 5–8 minutes or until softened and lightly browned. Stir in onion and sauté for another 5 minutes or until tender.
2. Add the sausage, sauerkraut, pepper, and salt. Cook uncovered over medium heat, until heated through, stirring continuously.

BACON-CABBAGE TOSS

TOTAL TIME: **45 minutes** | SERVES: **2 or 3**

5 slices turkey bacon, chopped

4 tablespoons ghee (clarified butter)

1 onion, chopped

½ head cabbage, shredded

1 teaspoon apple cider vinegar

sea salt and pepper

1. In a large skillet over medium heat, cook turkey bacon until crisp.
2. Add 2 tablespoons of the ghee. When melted, add onion and cook, stirring, until translucent.
3. Add cabbage and cook, stirring occasionally, until soft, 20–30 minutes.
4. Reduce heat to low and add vinegar and remaining 2 tablespoons ghee. Stir to combine and season with salt and pepper to taste.

Sides

KALE CHIPS

TOTAL TIME: **25 minutes** | SERVES: **2**

1 bunch kale, large stems removed and leaves roughly chopped

1 tablespoon fresh lemon juice

2 teaspoons coconut oil, melted

¼ teaspoon sea salt

1. Preheat oven to 350 degrees F. Line a baking sheet with parchment.
2. In a large bowl, combine all ingredients. Using hands, massage oil and seasonings onto kale until thoroughly coated.
3. Spread kale on prepared pan and bake until crisp, about 12 minutes.

Desserts

HOT CHOCOLATE SMOOTHIE

TOTAL TIME: **5 minutes** | SERVES: **1 or 2**

¼ cup coconut milk

¼ cup water

1 scoop chocolate protein powder or cocoa powder

2 tablespoons collagen powder

2 tablespoons chia seeds

stevia

1. Heat coconut milk and water in saucepan.
2. In a high-powered blender, combine all ingredients.
3. Puree on high until smooth.

Stressed Gut Recipes

These recipes are specifically designed to help support your adrenals, reduce your cortisol levels, and help your gut heal from the effects of stress.

Beverages & Breakfasts

BIRTHDAY CAKE SMOOTHIE

TOTAL TIME: **5 minutes** | SERVES: **1 or 2**

¾ cup coconut milk

1 banana

1 tablespoon coconut flour

1 tablespoon coconut butter, melted

1 tablespoon sprouted flaxseed

1 scoop protein powder

1 teaspoon vanilla extract

In a high-powered blender, combine all ingredients, sweetening with stevia to taste. Puree on high until smooth.

CHERRY PIE SMOOTHIE

TOTAL TIME: 5 minutes | SERVES: 1 or 2

½ cup frozen cherries

¼ cup coconut milk

½ teaspoon vanilla extract

¼ teaspoon cinnamon

pinch sea salt

pinch cardamom

stevia

Warm frozen cherries in saucepan. In a high-powered blender, combine all ingredients. Puree on high until smooth.

GOOD MORNING SMOOTHIE

TOTAL TIME: 5 minutes | SERVES: 1 or 2

½ cup goat's milk kefir or coconut milk

¼ cup blueberries

¼ cup blackberries

handful of chopped kale

1 scoop protein powder

1 tablespoon sprouted chia seeds

stevia

water

In a high-powered blender, combine all ingredients, sweetening with stevia to taste and adding water as necessary. Puree on high until smooth.

GI HEALING JUICE

TOTAL TIME: 5 minutes | SERVES: 1 or 2

½ head cabbage

1 cup aloe juice

1 cucumber

½ cup peppermint leaves

1 teaspoon grated fresh ginger

Add all ingredients to vegetable juicer. Gently stir juice and drink immediately.

PEAR PORRIDGE

TOTAL TIME: **10 minutes** | SERVES: **1**

1 pear, peeled and chopped	¼ teaspoon ginger powder
4 tablespoons coconut milk	1 scoop protein powder
2 tablespoons hemp seeds	stevia

1. In a blender, puree pear, coconut milk, hemp seeds, and ginger on high until smooth.
2. Pour into small saucepan over medium heat and warm through.
3. Remove from heat, stir in protein powder, and sweeten with stevia to taste. Transfer to bowl and serve warm.

Soups & Salads

APPLE-FENNEL SOUP

TOTAL TIME: **55 minutes** | SERVES: **4–6**

1 tablespoon coconut oil	2 cups cubed butternut squash
1 medium onion, sliced	1 knob fresh ginger, peeled and minced
1 bulb fennel, stalks removed, cored, and sliced	1 teaspoon sea salt
	1 teaspoon pepper
2 green apples, cored, peeled, and chopped	4 cups chicken bone broth

1. In a stockpot over medium heat, melt coconut oil. Add onion and cook, stirring occasionally, until starting to soften. Add fennel and apples and cook until slightly softened.
2. Add squash, ginger, salt, and pepper and stir to combine. Add broth, bring to a boil, and reduce heat to a simmer. Cook until vegetables are tender (the longer the simmering time, the more flavorful the soup).
3. Transfer soup to blender (or use immersion blender) and, working in batches if necessary, puree until smooth (be careful blending hot liquids). Return to pot, season to taste, and heat through.

CREAMY CUCUMBER-AVOCADO SOUP

TOTAL TIME: **10 minutes** | SERVES: **2–4**

5 ribs celery, halved crosswise

½ cucumber, peeled

1 avocado, halved and pitted

3 tablespoons fresh lemon juice

1 teaspoon sea salt

½ teaspoon pepper

½ cup water, divided

1. In a high-powered blender, combine celery and cucumber. Scoop avocado into blender. Add lemon juice, salt, pepper, and ¼ cup of the water.
2. Puree until smooth, adding the remaining ¼ cup water as necessary to reach desired consistency.

BLUEBERRY-BASIL KALE SALAD

TOTAL TIME: **20 minutes** | SERVES: **2 or 3**

DRESSING:

½ cup blueberries

¼ cup fresh basil leaves

2 tablespoons olive oil

5 teaspoons apple cider vinegar

1 teaspoon honey

sea salt

SALAD:

2 cups chopped kale

1–1½ cups chopped basil

3 cups cooked chicken

½ cup fresh blueberries

¼ cup chopped sprouted walnuts

½ cucumber, peeled and sliced

handful of sprouts

¼ red onion, chopped

1. To make the dressing: in a blender, combine blueberries, basil, oil, vinegar, and honey. Puree until smooth. Taste dressing, season with salt, and puree again to combine.
2. To prepare the salad: in a large bowl, combine all ingredients. Toss well.
3. Serve drizzled with dressing.

Main Dishes

SPAGHETTI SQUASH "ALFREDO"

TOTAL TIME: 1½ hours plus soaking time | SERVES: 4–6

1 cup raw cashews	⅛ teaspoon nutmeg
1 spaghetti squash	1 teaspoon fresh lemon juice
2 cups water	1 pound ground bison (or grass-fed
6 cloves garlic, minced	ground beef)
1 teaspoon sea salt	coconut oil

1. Soak cashews in water for 4 hours. Drain and set aside.
2. Preheat oven to 425 degrees F.
3. Prick squash all over with small sharp knife. Place on sheet pan and roast whole squash until tender when pierced with knife, 45–90 minutes, depending on size. Let cool.
4. In a blender, combine cashews and 2 cups water. Puree until a paste is formed. Add to small saucepan over medium heat with garlic, salt, and nutmeg. Cook until heated through. Stir in lemon juice. Keep warm.
5. In a skillet over medium-high heat, cook bison in coconut oil until no longer pink. Keep warm.
6. When squash is cool enough to handle, cut in half lengthwise and remove seeds with spoon. Use a fork to remove the "spaghetti" strands and place in serving bowl. Top with cooked bison and cashew sauce.

CHICKEN-AVOCADO BURGERS

TOTAL TIME: 25 minutes | SERVES: 4

1 pound ground chicken	1 clove garlic, minced
½ onion, chopped	1 avocado, halved and pitted
1 egg	sea salt and pepper
1 tablespoon chopped fresh parsley	coconut oil

1. In a bowl, combine chicken, onion, egg, parsley, and garlic. Scoop avocado into bowl. Season with salt and pepper. Mix well to combine and shape into 4 patties.

2. In a skillet over medium-high heat, cook patties in coconut oil, turning once, until no longer pink, 8–10 minutes.

BURRITO BOWL

TOTAL TIME: **5 minutes** | SERVES: **1**

1 cup shredded cooked chicken	shredded romaine lettuce
½ cup cooked kidney beans	no-added-sugar salsa
½ cup cooked black beans	guacamole

In a serving bowl, combine all ingredients and toss until well mixed.

TURKEY MEAT LOAF

TOTAL TIME: **1 hour** | SERVES: **4–6**

coconut oil	2 eggs
½ cup Mary's Gone Crackers crumbs, crushed	2 tablespoons coconut milk
2½ cups sun-dried tomatoes	2 cloves garlic, minced
½ cup goat cheese (chèvre)	2 teaspoons sea salt
⅓ cup chopped fresh parsley	1 teaspoon pepper
	1 pound ground turkey

1. Preheat oven to 375 degrees F. Grease a 9 x 5–inch loaf pan with coconut oil.

2. In a large bowl, combine cracker crumbs, sun-dried tomatoes, cheese, parsley, eggs, coconut milk, garlic, salt, and pepper. Add turkey and mix well.

3. Pack mixture into prepared pan and bake until cooked through and no longer pink, about 45 minutes.

Sides

BAKED VEGETABLE FRIES

TOTAL TIME: **55 minutes** | SERVES: **2–4**

1 rutabaga, peeled

2–3 carrots

1 red bell pepper, seeded and ribs
    removed

1 onion

2 portobello mushroom caps

1–2 tablespoons coconut oil, melted

2 teaspoons onion powder

2 teaspoons garlic powder

sea salt and pepper

1. Preheat oven to 425 degrees F.
2. Cut vegetables into long, thin strips (you should have about a cup of each)
3. Place on large baking sheet (working in batches if necessary) and toss with coconut oil to coat. Spread in single layer, sprinkle with onion powder and garlic powder, and season with salt and pepper.
4. Roast until vegetables are tender and golden brown, about 40 minutes.

Desserts

PEPPERMINT PATTIES

TOTAL TIME: **30 minutes plus chilling time** | SERVES: **12**

2 cups coconut oil, at room
    temperature

½ cup honey

1 teaspoon peppermint extract

3 dark chocolate bars (3 ounces each),
    minimum 72 percent cacao

½ cup coconut oil, melted

1. In a bowl, mix first three ingredients. Form into small patties, set on plate lined with parchment, and place in freezer to harden.
2. Meanwhile, in a saucepan over medium-low heat, melt chocolate and the remaining ½ cup coconut oil. Remove from heat and let cool for 5–10 minutes.
3. Dip the hardened patties into the chocolate mixture until covered and return to parchment. Freeze until chocolate hardens. Store in refrigerator or freezer.

Immune Gut Recipes

These recipes are specifically designed to help tamp down inflammation, manage food sensitivities, and attempt to interrupt the autoimmune cycle. (Note: while these recipes do not feature many of the most common allergens, please review every recipe for any foods that may cause issues for you.)

Beverages & Breakfasts

CINNAMON BUN SMOOTHIE RECIPE

TOTAL TIME: **5 minutes** | SERVES: **1 or 2**

1 cup coconut milk

1 banana

1 tablespoon sprouted flaxseed

1 teaspoon pure maple syrup

1 tablespoon collagen powder

1 teaspoon vanilla extract

¾ teaspoon cinnamon

In a high-powered blender, combine all ingredients. Puree on high until smooth.

BAKED APPLE SMOOTHIE

TOTAL TIME: **5 minutes** | SERVES: **1 or 2**

1 apple, cored and seeded

¼ cup coconut milk

1 tablespoon flax meal

2 tablespoon vanilla protein or
   collagen powder

½ teaspoon cinnamon

½ teaspoon vanilla extract

pinch ginger

stevia

1. Bake apple in roasting pan in oven at 350 degrees F for 30 minutes.
2. In a high-powered blender, combine the baked apple and remaining ingredients, sweetening with stevia to taste. Puree on high until smooth.

MANGO-STRAWBERRY SMOOTHIE

TOTAL TIME: 5 minutes | SERVES: 1 or 2

½ cup mango chunks   ½ cup strawberries
½ cup coconut milk   ½ cucumber, peeled
½ cup coconut water   stevia

In a high-powered blender, combine all ingredients, sweetening with stevia to taste. Puree on high until smooth.

COCONUT FLOUR BLUEBERRY MUFFINS

TOTAL TIME: 30 minutes | SERVES: 12

12 egg yolks   1 teaspoon baking powder
6 tablespoons coconut oil, melted   ½ cup coconut flour
3 tablespoons coconut sugar   1 cup fresh blueberries
1 tablespoon vanilla   stevia to taste
½ teaspoon sea salt

1. Preheat oven to 400 degrees F and line muffin tins.
2. Mix all ingredients in a bowl until well combined.
3. Pour batter into lined muffin tins. Bake for 14–20 minutes or until cooked through, testing for doneness.

Soups & Salads

BERRY SOUP

TOTAL TIME: 10 minutes | SERVES: 1

½ cup blueberries   ¼ cup fresh lime juice
½ cup strawberries   1 scoop protein powder
1 cucumber, peeled

1. In a saucepan over medium heat, warm berries.
2. Puree in a high-powered blender with remaining ingredients and serve.

SLOW-COOKER LEMONGRASS-CHICKEN SOUP

TOTAL TIME: 6½ hours | SERVES: 4

1 pound boneless, skinless chicken
  breasts
3 cups chicken bone broth
2 cups chopped cabbage
1 cup sliced mushrooms
4 carrots, chopped
⅓ cup sliced onion

¼ cup fresh lemon juice
2 stalks lemongrass, smashed, or zest
  of 1 lemon, cut into strips
4 cloves garlic, minced
1 small knob fresh ginger, peeled and
  minced
sea salt

1. In a slow cooker, combine all ingredients. Cook on low for 6–8 hours.
2. Remove and discard lemongrass or lemon zest. Remove chicken breasts from slow cooker and chop up. Then add back into the pot and stir to distribute before serving. Season with salt to taste.

Main Dishes

SLOW-COOKER BEEF AND BROCCOLI

TOTAL TIME: 6¼ hours | SERVES: 2 or 3

¼ cup coconut aminos (a soy sauce
  alternative)
¼ cup beef bone broth
2 tablespoons apple cider vinegar
2 teaspoons coconut oil, melted

4 cloves garlic, minced
¼ teaspoon crushed red-pepper flakes
sea salt and pepper
1 pound grass-fed steak, cut into strips
1 head broccoli, cut into florets

1. In a slow cooker, combine coconut aminos, broth, vinegar, and coconut oil. Stir in garlic and red-pepper flakes and season with salt and pepper. Add beef and stir to coat. Add broccoli and stir again.
2. Cook on low for 6 hours.

GRILLED HONEY-GLAZED SALMON

TOTAL TIME: **20 minutes** | SERVES: **4**

¼ cup honey

¼ cup coconut aminos (a soy sauce alternative)

4 cloves garlic, minced

1 tablespoon ghee (clarified butter), melted

1 tablespoon fresh thyme leaves

1 teaspoon grated or minced fresh ginger

sea salt and pepper

2 pounds wild-caught Alaskan salmon fillets

coconut oil

1. In a shallow baking dish, whisk together honey, coconut aminos, garlic, ghee, thyme, and ginger. Season with salt and pepper.
2. Place salmon in baking dish and coat with mixture. Chill for 15 minutes, turn fish to coat other side, and chill another 15 minutes.
3. Prepare lightly oiled (with coconut oil) grill for medium heat.
4. Shake off excess marinade from salmon and discard. Grill until fish flakes easily with a fork, 5–8 minutes per side.

BISON BURGERS

TOTAL TIME: **20 minutes** | SERVES: **4**

1 pound ground bison (or grass-fed ground beef)

1 tablespoon garlic powder

1 tablespoon Worcestershire sauce

2 teaspoons sea salt

2 teaspoons pepper

2 teaspoons onion powder

½ teaspoon cumin

coconut oil

3–4 cups fresh or cooked spinach

1. In a large bowl, combine all ingredients except coconut oil and spinach. Mix thoroughly and form into four patties.
2. In a skillet over medium-high heat, cook patties in coconut oil, turning once, 8–12 minutes or until desired doneness.
3. Serve over a bed of spinach.

AVOCADO–TUNA SALAD LETTUCE WRAPS

TOTAL TIME: 15 minutes | SERVES: 1 or 2

1 can (5–6 ounces) wild-caught tuna
½ avocado, halved and pitted
¼ onion, chopped
1 tablespoon chopped fresh parsley
2 teaspoons fresh lemon juice

1 teaspoon sea salt
pepper
1 teaspoon olive oil
romaine lettuce leaves

1. Flake tuna into bowl. Scoop avocado out of peel and add to bowl. Add onion, parsley, lemon juice, salt, pepper, and oil and mix well.
2. Serve tuna salad in romaine leaves.

Sides

CHARD GREENS

TOTAL TIME: 1½ hours | SERVES: 4–6

1 tablespoon coconut oil
2 tablespoons garlic, minced
5 cups chicken bone broth

5 bunches chard, trimmed and
  chopped
sea salt and pepper

1. In a large pot over medium heat, melt coconut oil. Add garlic and cook, stirring, for 2–3 minutes. Pour in broth and bring to a boil. Reduce heat and simmer for 30 minutes.
2. Add chard and raise heat to medium-high. Let greens cook down for about 45 minutes, stirring occasionally.
3. Reduce heat to medium and cook until greens are tender. Season with salt and pepper to taste.

Desserts

FRUIT SNACKS

TOTAL TIME: 15 minutes plus chilling time | SERVES: Varies

⅔ cup fresh lime juice

⅔ cup blueberries

stevia

5 tablespoons unflavored gelatin (or vegan substitute, such as agar-agar or carrageenan)

1. In a small saucepan over medium heat, combine lime juice and blueberries. Cook, stirring occasionally, until berries soften.
2. Sweeten with stevia to taste, stirring until well incorporated.
3. Transfer to blender and puree until smooth. Gradually add gelatin 1 tablespoon at a time with blender running. Blend continuously for 5 minutes.
4. Pour into an 8-inch (or smaller) square baking dish (or use ice cube molds). Chill until set, at least 1 hour, and cut as desired.

Gastric Gut Recipes

These recipes are specifically designed to help stop acid reflux and improve digestion. (Note: as delicious as these recipes are, please remember to take your time and chew every bite thirty times to allow your digestive enzymes to do their work thoroughly.)

Beverages & Breakfasts

MORNING GLORY SMOOTHIE

TOTAL TIME: 5 minutes | SERVES: 1 or 2

1 cup mango chunks

1 cup goat's milk kefir

½ cup strawberries

½ cucumber, peeled

stevia

In a high-powered blender, combine all ingredients, sweetening with stevia to taste. Puree on high until smooth.

PIÑA COLADA SMOOTHIE

TOTAL TIME: 5 minutes | SERVES: 1 or 2

1 cup coconut milk

½ cup frozen pineapple

½ banana

¼ cup protein powder

3 tablespoons sprouted chia seeds

1 tablespoon honey

1 teaspoon coconut oil, melted

½ teaspoon vanilla extract

In a high-powered blender, combine all ingredients. Puree on high until smooth.

STOMACH-SOOTHING SMOOTHIE

TOTAL TIME: 5 minutes | SERVES: 1 or 2

1 cup coconut water

½ cup aloe vera juice

1 cucumber, peeled

½ green apple, peeled

1 scoop protein powder

In a high-powered blender, combine all ingredients. Puree on high until smooth.

TURMERIC TEA RECIPE

TOTAL TIME: 5 minutes | SERVES: 1 or 2

1 cup coconut milk

1 cup water

1 tablespoon ghee (clarified butter)

1 teaspoon turmeric

stevia

1. In a small saucepan over medium heat, combine coconut milk and water. Warm through, about 2 minutes.
2. Stir in ghee, turmeric, and stevia to taste. Cook, stirring, until heated through, about 2 minutes longer.

HOMEMADE GRANOLA

TOTAL TIME: **45 minutes** | SERVES: **16–20**

½ cup coconut oil plus additional for greasing pan

3 cups gluten-free oats

2 cups shredded unsweetened coconut

2 cups sliced almonds

½ cup honey

1 cup dried cranberries

1 cup dried apricots, chopped

1. Preheat oven to 350 degrees F. Grease sheet pan with coconut oil.
2. In a large bowl, toss together oats, coconut, almonds, and honey.
3. Spread granola on sheet pan. Bake, stirring occasionally, until golden brown, 30–45 minutes, watching carefully not to burn. Remove granola from oven and let cool. Stir in cranberries and apricots. Transfer to airtight storage containers.

Soups & Salads

ONION SOUP

TOTAL TIME: **50 minutes** | SERVES: **4–6**

2 tablespoons ghee (clarified butter)

4 large onions, thinly sliced

2 cups chicken bone broth

2 cups beef bone broth

5 cloves garlic, chopped

sea salt and pepper

1. In a stockpot over medium heat, melt ghee. Add onions and cook, stirring occasionally, until lightly caramelized.
2. Add broths and garlic. Season with salt and pepper to taste.
3. Bring mixture to a boil, reduce heat, and simmer for 30–50 minutes (the longer the simmering time, the more flavorful the soup).

MUSHROOM SOUP

TOTAL TIME: 45 minutes | SERVES: 2–4

2–3 tablespoons ghee (clarified butter)
1 cup chopped onion
3 cups mushrooms, trimmed and sliced
1½ teaspoons paprika
1½ teaspoons coconut aminos (a soy sauce alternative)
1 teaspoon dillweed

1 cup chicken bone broth
½ cup coconut milk
1½ tablespoons arrowroot powder
2 tablespoons chopped fresh parsley
1 teaspoon apple cider vinegar
½ teaspoon sea salt
½ teaspoon pepper

1. In a large pot over medium heat, melt ghee. Add onion and cook, stirring occasionally, 5 minutes. Add mushrooms and cook, stirring occasionally, for another 5 minutes. Stir in paprika, coconut aminos, and dillweed. Add broth.
2. In a small bowl, whisk together coconut milk and arrowroot powder. Add to pot and stir well to blend. Cover and simmer 15 minutes, stirring occasionally.
3. Stir in parsley, vinegar, salt, and pepper. Warm through over low heat for 3–5 minutes.

BONE BROTH CHICKEN VEGETABLE SOUP

TOTAL TIME: 6½ hours | SERVES: 4–6

3 or 4 boneless, skinless chicken breasts
4 cups chicken bone broth
5 ribs celery, chopped
5 carrots, chopped

1 onion, chopped
4 cloves garlic, minced
4 thyme sprigs
sea salt and pepper
1 tablespoon chopped fresh parsley

1. In a slow cooker, combine all ingredients but the parsley. Cook on low for 6 hours.
2. Using slotted spoon, remove chicken and chop up before adding back into the mixture. Taste and adjust seasoning if necessary. Serve topped with parsley.

Main Dishes

LAMB BURGERS

TOTAL TIME: **30 minutes** | SERVES: **4**

1 pound ground lamb

½ onion, chopped

2 tablespoons fresh lemon juice

1 tablespoon chopped fresh dill

1 tablespoon chopped fresh mint leaves

2 teaspoons chopped fresh oregano

sea salt

coconut oil

3–4 cups fresh or cooked spinach

1. In a bowl, combine lamb, onion, lemon juice, and herbs. Season with salt. Mix until seasonings are evenly dispersed through meat. Form into four patties.
2. In a skillet over medium-high heat, cook patties in coconut oil, turning once, until no longer pink, 8–12 minutes.
3. Serve over a bed of spinach.

BAKED ARTICHOKE CHICKEN

TOTAL TIME: **1 hour** | SERVES: **4**

1–2 tablespoons ghee (clarified butter), plus additional for greasing pan

1 onion, chopped

1 cup sliced mushrooms

garlic powder

Italian seasoning

sea salt and pepper

8 ounces goat cheese (chèvre)

½ cup chicken bone broth

1 can (14 ounces) artichoke hearts, drained

1 cup fresh spinach

4 boneless, skinless chicken breasts

1. Preheat oven to 350 degrees F. Lightly grease a 13 x 9–inch baking pan with ghee.
2. In a skillet over medium heat, cook onion in ghee, stirring occasionally, until softened. Add mushrooms and cook until golden. Season with garlic powder, Italian seasoning, and salt and pepper to taste.
3. Crumble goat cheese into pan, add broth, and stir well to combine. Stir in artichoke hearts and spinach.

4. Put chicken in prepared baking pan. Pour artichoke mixture over top and bake until chicken is cooked through, about 30 minutes.

BAKED GROUPER WITH COCONUT-CILANTRO SAUCE

TOTAL TIME: 30 minutes | SERVES: 4

2 tablespoons coconut oil

4 wild-caught grouper fillets (6 ounces each)

¼ teaspoon sea salt

½ cup coconut milk

½ cup cilantro leaves

2 cloves garlic, minced

1 teaspoon minced fresh ginger

½ teaspoon curry powder

1. Preheat oven to 425 degrees F. Grease a 13 x 9–inch baking pan with coconut oil.

2. Place fish in the prepared pan. Sprinkle with salt.

3. Combine coconut milk, cilantro, garlic, ginger, and curry powder in a food processor. Pulse until smooth. Pour half of the mixture over fish. Bake until fish flakes easily, 15–20 minutes.

4. Pour remaining mixture over baked fish and serve.

Sides

FRIED "FAUX" RICE

TOTAL TIME: 20 minutes | SERVES: 3 or 4

1 large head broccoli, chopped into small florets

3½ tablespoons ghee (clarified butter), divided

1 onion, chopped

1 carrot, shredded

sea salt and pepper

2 eggs, lightly beaten

2 tablespoons coconut aminos (a soy sauce alternative)

1. In a high-powered blender, pulse broccoli until it resembles grains of rice, being careful not to overprocess.

2. In a skillet over medium heat, cook "riced" broccoli with onion and carrot in 3 tablespoons of the ghee, stirring occasionally, until tender. Season with salt and pepper to taste. Keep warm.

(*continued on next page*)

3. In another skillet over medium heat, melt remaining ½ tablespoon ghee. Add eggs and stir to scramble them and chop finely. Immediately add to broccoli mixture and stir to combine.

4. Stir in coconut aminos, warm through, and serve immediately.

Desserts

RAW VANILLA ICE CREAM

TOTAL TIME: 10 minutes plus soaking/freezing time | SERVES: 2

2 cups raw cashews

2 cups coconut meat

1 cup honey

⅓ cup coconut butter

2 tablespoons vanilla extract

½ teaspoon sea salt

¾ cup water (as needed)

1. Soak cashews in water for 4 hours. Drain and set aside.

2. In a blender, combine coconut meat, honey, coconut butter, vanilla extract, and salt. Puree until smooth and creamy, adding water as needed to keep mixture circulating in blender.

3. Once mixed well, add the drained cashews and blend until smooth and whipped.

4. Transfer mixture to a bowl and freeze until desired consistency is reached.

Toxic Gut Recipes

These recipes are specifically designed to support the liver and gallbladder and help your body digest fats effectively, as well as soothe emotional discord and decrease stress.

Beverages & Breakfasts

CHOCOLATE-COVERED STRAWBERRY SMOOTHIE

TOTAL TIME: 5 minutes | SERVES: 1 or 2

1 cup frozen strawberries
½ cup goat's milk kefir or yogurt
½ cup coconut water

1 tablespoon raw cacao
1 scoop chocolate protein powder
stevia

In a high-powered blender, combine all ingredients. Puree on high until smooth.

OMEGA BLUEBERRY SMOOTHIE

TOTAL TIME: 5 minutes | SERVES: 1 or 2

1 cup blueberries
¼ cup goat's milk kefir
½ cup coconut water

1 tablespoon sprouted flaxseed
1 scoop vanilla protein powder

In a high-powered blender, combine all ingredients. Puree on high until smooth.

WAKE-ME-UP SMOOTHIE

TOTAL TIME: 5 minutes | SERVES: 1 or 2

½ cucumber, peeled
½ green apple, peeled and cored
½ cup fresh pineapple cubes
½ cup goat's milk kefir

1 tablespoon sprouted chia seeds
1 scoop protein powder
1 teaspoon honey
water (as needed)

In a high-powered blender, combine all ingredients, adding water as necessary. Puree on high until smooth.

BREAKFAST WRAP

TOTAL TIME: **10 minutes** | SERVES: **1**

coconut oil

2 or 3 eggs

sea salt and pepper

½ cup kimchi

¼ cup shredded cooked chicken breast

1 slice turkey bacon, cooked

handful of sprouts

1 Ezekiel 4:9 Sprouted Whole Grain
  Tortilla

1. In small skillet over medium heat, cook eggs in coconut oil. Season with salt and pepper to taste.
2. Put eggs, kimchi, chicken, turkey bacon, and sprouts on tortilla, wrap to enclose fillings, and serve.

Soups & Salads

BUTTERNUT SQUASH—BACON SOUP

TOTAL TIME: **45 minutes** | SERVES: **8**

2–3 tablespoons coconut oil

2 onions, finely chopped

3 cloves garlic, minced

16 strips turkey bacon, chopped

4 cups butternut squash (cooked or
  canned)

5–7 cups chicken bone broth

1 cup coconut milk

sea salt and pepper

1. In a stockpot over medium heat, cook onions in coconut oil, stirring occasionally, until translucent. Add garlic and turkey bacon to stockpot, then cook, stirring, until fragrant.
2. Stir in squash and add broth and coconut milk to reach desired consistency. Bring to a boil, reduce heat, and simmer until slightly reduced, about 30 minutes. Season with salt and pepper to taste.

BEET AND POMEGRANATE SALAD

TOTAL TIME: 1¼ hours | SERVES: 2 or 3

3 beets with tops trimmed to 1 inch

1 cup diced red onion

¼ cup coconut vinegar

¼ cup chicken bone broth

3 tablespoons grated orange zest

1 tablespoon pure maple syrup

sea salt

1 cup pomegranate seeds

2 cups spinach and arugula leaves

¼ cup crumbled raw goat cheese

1. Preheat oven to 400 degrees F. Wrap beets tightly in heavy-duty foil.
2. Roast beets until tender, 50–60 minutes. Cool, peel, and cut into cubes.
3. In a saucepan over medium heat, bring beets, onion, vinegar, broth, orange zest, and maple syrup to a boil, stirring often. After 5 minutes, remove from heat and cool to room temperature. Season with salt to taste.
4. Stir pomegranate seeds into beet mixture. Serve over salad greens and top with cheese.

SUPERFOOD SALAD

TOTAL TIME: 10 minutes | SERVES: 1

1 cup fresh spinach

½ cup chopped cooked chicken breast

½ cup chopped cooked beets

½ green apple, cored and chopped

¼ cup sprouted chia seeds

handful of sprouts

1 tablespoon olive oil

1 tablespoon balsamic vinegar

½ teaspoon fresh lemon juice

1. In a serving bowl, combine spinach, chicken, beets, apple, chia seeds, and sprouts, as desired.
2. Drizzle oil, vinegar, and lemon juice over top and toss to coat well.

Main Dishes

GARLIC BAKED CHICKEN

TOTAL TIME: **30 minutes** | SERVES: **2**

1 tablespoon coconut oil, melted, plus
    additional for greasing pan
2 boneless, skinless chicken breasts
½ onion, finely chopped
¼ cup seedless raisins
3–6 cloves garlic, minced

2 teaspoons dried rosemary
1½ teaspoons chopped fresh parsley
½ teaspoon cinnamon
½ teaspoon sea salt
½ teaspoon pepper

1. Preheat oven to 450 degrees F.
2. Line a baking pan with parchment and grease with coconut oil. Place chicken on parchment.
3. In a bowl, combine remaining ingredients and mix well. Spread onto chicken.
4. Bake until chicken is cooked through, 20–25 minutes.

LETTUCE-WRAPPED TURKEY SLOPPY JOES

TOTAL TIME: **20 minutes** | SERVES: **4**

coconut oil
1 pound ground turkey
½ onion, chopped
½ bell pepper, chopped

1 recipe Dr. Axe's Sweet & Tangy
    Barbecue Sauce (see below)
16 Bibb lettuce leaves (4 per burger)
1 cup sauerkraut

1. In a medium skillet over medium-high heat, cook turkey in coconut oil, breaking up clumps, until no longer pink.
2. Add onion and pepper and cook, stirring, until softened. Stir in barbecue sauce.
3. Serve turkey mixture in lettuce leaves and top with sauerkraut.

DR. AXE'S SWEET & TANGY BARBECUE SAUCE

TOTAL TIME: 55 minutes | SERVES: 10–15

2 cups organic tomato sauce

½ cup water

½ cup balsamic vinegar

⅓ cup honey

¼ cup coconut aminos

1 tablespoon stone-ground mustard

1½ teaspoons onion powder

1½ teaspoons garlic powder

½ teaspoon sea salt

1. In a high-powered blender, combine all ingredients and puree until smooth.
2. Transfer to a medium saucepan and bring to a boil over medium-high heat. Reduce heat and simmer for 45 minutes.
3. Store extra sauce in the refrigerator.

SALMON PATTIES

TOTAL TIME: 20 minutes | SERVES: 1 or 2

1 can (6–7 ounces) wild-caught Alaskan salmon, drained

2 eggs

¼ box Mary's Gone Crackers, crumbled

¼ onion, chopped

½ teaspoon dillweed

½ teaspoon sea salt

1 tablespoon coconut oil

1. In a medium bowl, combine salmon, eggs, crackers, onion, dillweed, and salt. Mix with hands to combine. Form into patties.
2. In a skillet over medium-high heat, cook patties in coconut oil, turning once, until golden brown and heated through, 8–10 minutes.

Vegan Leaky Gut Recipes

These recipes combine all of the benefits of the other recipes while avoiding all animal products. (Note: feel free to experiment with vegan versions of any recipe in the Eat Dirt recipes—many taste just as delicious without meat!)

Beverages & Breakfasts

GREEN PROTEIN SMOOTHIE

TOTAL TIME: 5 minutes | SERVES: 1 or 2

½ bunch spinach

½ banana

½ cucumber, peeled

½ avocado

½ cup ice

1 teaspoon cinnamon

½ cup coconut milk

water (as needed)

Place all ingredients in a blender and blend on high until well incorporated.

RASPBERRY-BANANA-CHIA SMOOTHIE

TOTAL TIME: 5 minutes | SERVES: 1 or 2

1 cup raspberries

1 banana

1 cup coconut milk

1 teaspoon maple syrup

1 tablespoon sprouted flaxseeds

1 tablespoon sprouted chia seeds

Place all ingredients in a blender and blend on high until desired consistency is reached.

SWEET POTATO—BEET HASH

TOTAL TIME: 45 minutes | SERVES: 2–4

1 large sweet potato, peeled and cubed

1 large beet, peeled and cubed

1 tablespoon coconut oil, melted

1 teaspoon salt, plus additional for
    seasoning

½ teaspoon pepper

1 onion, diced

1. Preheat oven to 400 degrees F. Toss sweet potato and beet with coconut oil and season with salt and pepper.
2. Place on a baking sheet and bake for 25–30 minutes until cooked through.
3. In a skillet over medium heat, add onion and season with salt. Cook until onions caramelize.

4. Add the sweet potatoes and beets to the pan and stir. Cook for another 5 minutes.

BAKED QUINOA WITH APPLES

TOTAL TIME: **25 minutes** | SERVES: **1**

½ cup quinoa, rinsed

2 tablespoons sprouted flaxseed mixed
   in 6 tablespoons of water

5 tablespoons applesauce

⅛ teaspoon sea salt

¼ teaspoon cinnamon

2 tablespoons pecans, chopped

¾ cup apple, chopped

1 teaspoon maple syrup

1. Cook quinoa as indicated on package.

2. Pour quinoa into oven-safe bowl. Add flaxseed and water mixture, applesauce, salt, and cinnamon. Broil in oven on low for 7 minutes.

3. Top with pecans, apple, and maple syrup.

Soups & Salads

VEGAN APPLE-FENNEL SOUP

TOTAL TIME: **55 minutes** | SERVES: **4–6**

1 tablespoon coconut oil

1 medium onion, sliced

1 bulb fennel, stalks removed, cored,
   and sliced

2 green apples, cored, peeled, and
   chopped

2 cups cubed butternut squash

1 knob fresh ginger, peeled and minced

1 teaspoon sea salt

1 teaspoon pepper

4 cups vegetable broth

1. In a stockpot over medium heat, melt coconut oil. Add onion and cook, stirring occasionally, until starting to soften. Add fennel and apples and cook until slightly softened.

2. Add squash, ginger, salt, and pepper and stir to combine. Add broth, bring to a boil, and reduce heat to a simmer. Cook until vegetables are tender (the longer the simmering time, the more flavorful the soup).

3. Transfer soup to blender (or use immersion blender) and, working in batches if necessary, puree until smooth (be careful blending hot liquids). Return to pot, season to taste, and heat through.

CABBAGE SALAD

TOTAL TIME: 40 minutes | SERVES: 1 or 2

2 tablespoons coconut oil

1 onion, chopped

½ head cabbage, shredded

½ cup pine nuts

4 tablespoons coconut oil

1 teaspoon apple cider vinegar

1 teaspoon sea salt

½ teaspoon pepper

1. Add coconut oil and the onion to a skillet over medium-high heat and cook until translucent.
2. Add cabbage and cook until soft, about 20–30 minutes.
3. Turn heat to low and add remaining ingredients. Mix until well incorporated.

ARTICHOKE SOUP

TOTAL TIME: 15 minutes | SERVES: 1

2 tablespoons coconut oil

1 onion, chopped

1 cup mushrooms

1 cup vegetable broth

½ teaspoon garlic powder

1 teaspoon sea salt

½ teaspoon pepper

1 teaspoon Italian seasoning

1 can artichoke hearts

1 cup spinach

1. Add coconut oil, onion, and mushrooms to a skillet over medium-high heat and cook until softened.
2. In a pot over medium heat, heat broth. Add spices, artichokes, spinach, and onion and mushroom mixture. Cook until heated and cooked through.

Main Dishes

SLOW-COOKER VEGETABLE SOUP

TOTAL TIME: 6–8 hours | SERVES: 4–6

4 sweet potatoes, peeled

3 carrots, peeled

3 onions

3 cups mushrooms, chopped

1 cup uncooked quinoa

1 teaspoon sea salt

½ teaspoon pepper

¾ teaspoon poultry seasoning

1½ tablespoons Worcestershire sauce

5 cups vegetable broth

1. Dice potatoes, carrots, and onions into medium-sized chunks.
2. Place vegetables and remaining ingredients in slow cooker and mix well.
3. Cook on low for 6–8 hours or until cooked through. Adjust seasoning as needed.

SAUTÉED PESTO SPAGHETTI SQUASH

TOTAL TIME: 1¾ hours | SERVES: 2

1 spaghetti squash

2 cups fresh basil, sage, cilantro, and parsley

2 garlic cloves, chopped

½ cup olive oil

¼ cup pine nuts

2 tablespoons coconut oil

2 cups fresh mushrooms, sliced

1. Preheat oven to 425 degrees F. Poke spaghetti squash with fork numerous times and place in a pan. Bake in oven for 45 minutes to 1½ hours, depending on size. (Poke with a fork; it should be soft when cooked through.)
2. After squash is cooked, remove from oven. Once it has cooled, cut it in half lengthwise.
3. Remove the flesh with a spoon, then with a fork, comb against the "spaghetti" strands to piece them apart and remove from skin.
4. Make pesto by combining herbs, garlic, olive oil, and pine nuts in a food processor and process until the mixture is creamy.
5. In a skillet over medium-high heat with coconut oil, sauté mushrooms until softened. Add mushrooms and pesto on top of spaghetti squash and serve.

EZEKIEL WRAP

TOTAL TIME: 5 minutes | SERVES: 1

2 tablespoons hummus

1 Ezekiel 4:9 Sprouted Whole Grain
   Tortilla (if gluten intolerant, use
   coconut or rice wrap)

4 ounces mushrooms

½ cup sprouts

½ avocado, chopped

½ cup sauerkraut

1. Using a spoon, spread the hummus over the wrap evenly.
2. Layer on the mushrooms, sprouts, avocado, and sauerkraut.
3. Fold the wrap to hold everything in place.

Desserts

BLUEBERRY PUDDING

TOTAL TIME: 5 minutes | SERVES: 4–6

1 cup coconut milk

1 cup kefir

3 avocados

1 cup blueberries

4 tablespoons sprouted chia seeds,
   ground

½ teaspoon sea salt

1 tablespoon vanilla

1 drop peppermint oil extract

1 tablespoon honey

Place all ingredients in a high-powered blender and blend on high until
well incorporated.

Resource Guide

Dr. Axe Community and Support

- ▶ Dr. Josh Axe's website: www.draxe.com
- ▶ Facebook: www.facebook.com/drjoshaxe
- ▶ Pinterest: www.pinterest.com/draxe
- ▶ YouTube: www.youtube.com/doctorjoshaxe

Supplements

- ▶ Axe Organics: www.store.draxe.com
- ▶ Numa Essentials: www.NumaEssentials.com
- ▶ Probiome RX: www.ProBiomeRX.com
- ▶ Doctor Collagen: www.DoctorCollagen.com
- ▶ Get Real: www.GetRealNutrition.com

Organic Food

- ▶ Axe Nutrition products: www.store.draxe.com/food
- ▶ Bone broth: www.wisechoicemarket.com
- ▶ Sprouted grains: www.healthyflour.com
- ▶ Wild seafood: www.vitalchoice.com
- ▶ Organic snacks: www.thrivemarket.com

Essential Oils

- ▶ Numa Essentials: www.NumaEssentials.com

Kitchen Equipment

▸ To find everything from slow cookers to blenders and water filters to cookware, check out the products Dr. Axe personally uses and recommends at: www.draxe.com/resources

Lab Testing

▸ 23andMe: www.23andme.com
▸ Great Plains: www.greatplainslaboratory.com
▸ Genova Diagnostics: www.gdx.net
▸ uBiome: www.ubiome.com

Bonus Gifts

▸ Essential oils eBook: www.draxe.com/essential-oils-book-bonus
▸ Replacement food list: www.draxe.com/replacement-food-list
▸ Mom's daily plan: www.draxe.com/healing-plan-bonus
▸ Guide to eating out: www.draxe.com/eating-out-guide
▸ Smoothie recipe eBook: www.draxe.com/smoothie-guide -bonus
▸ Shopping list: www.draxe.com/eat-dirt-shopping-list
▸ Leaky gut top-25 supplement guide: www.draxe.com/leaky -gut-supplements-bonus
▸ Bonus interviews with guest experts: www.draxe.com/eat -dirt-bonus-interviews

Acknowledgments

I first want to thank God, my lord and savior Jesus Christ, for loving me and giving me the opportunity, the influence, and the gifts to write this book.

To my wife, Chelsea, you are the light of my life and I couldn't have written this book without you. Your wisdom and love make me a better man, leader, and teacher.

To my agent, Bonnie Solow, you are the best literary agent on the planet and I have been so blessed by your advice and pursuit of excellence.

To my editor, Julie Will, whose insight, patience, and skill helped make this book great. And special thanks to the whole HarperWave team: Karen Rinaldi, Brian Perrin, Victoria Comella, and Kate Lyons.

To my PR team at DunnPellier Media, including Nicole Dunn. Thank you for helping spread this message and believing in me early on.

To Mariska van Aalst, for helping create a masterpiece.

To the DrAxe.com team, including Evan, Mike, Ethan, Juliana, and Mary, I could not do this alone and it takes not only a team, but a passionate team of A players to change the world.

To my friends who are health leaders, including: Jordan Rubin, JJ Virgin, Sara Gottfried, Vani Hari, Leanne Ely, Donna Gates, Mark Hyman, David Perlmutter, Eric Zielinski, Sayer Ji, Izabella Wentz, Alan Christianson, Brian Mowll, Peter Osborne, Kelly Brogan, Ty Bollinger, Steven Masley, Amy Myers, Yuri Elkaim, Tom O'Bryan, Cynthia Pasquella, Robin Openshaw, Lewis Howes and Pete Camiolo. Thanks for supporting this book and helping transform the health of a nation.

To my parents, Gary and Winona Axe. Thank you for raising me in a loving home and always encouraging me. Dad, you taught me discipline, humility, and the importance of doing plenty of pull-ups. And, Mom, you are the most courageous person I know and taught me the importance of prayer and persistence.

To my in-laws, Joel and Sherri Vreeman. Thank you for all of your love and support, and for being an example of how to be a light to the world.

To Axe Nation and the Axe Ambassadors, thank you for passionately helping spread this message of health and natural healing.

And finally, to my dog, Oakley, thanks for teaching me every day that dirt is my friend.

Notes

INTRODUCTION

1. Dabelea, D., et al. SEARCH for Diabetes in Youth Study. "Prevalence of type 1 and type 2 diabetes among children and adolescents from 2001 to 2009." *JAMA*. 2014, May 7; 311(17):1778–86.
2. www.aarda.org/autoimmune-information/autoimmune-statistics.
3. www.niddk.nih.gov/health-information/health-statistics/Pages/overweight-obesity-statistics.aspx.
4. www.foodallergy.org/facts-and-stats.
5. www.ccfa.org/assets/pdfs/updatedibdfactbook.pdf.
6. www.aarda.org/autoimmune-information/autoimmune-statistics.
7. www.liverfoundation.org/chapters/lam2010.

CHAPTER 1

1. Hadhazy, A. "Think Twice: How the Gut's Second Brain Influences Mood and Well-being." 2010, Feb 12. *Scientific American*. www.scientificamerican.com/article/gut-second-brain.
2. www.nih.gov/news-events/news-releases/nih-human-microbiome-project-de fines-normal-bacterial-makeup-body.
3. Martín, R., et al. "Role of commensal and probiotic bacteria in human health: a focus on inflammatory bowel disease." *Microb Cell Fact*. 2013, July 23; 12:71.
4. http://draxe.com/probiotics-benefits-foods-supplements.
5. Arrieta, M. C., et al. "Alterations in Intestinal Permeability." *Gut*. 2006, Oct; 55(10):1512–20; www.ncbi.nlm.nih.gov/pmc/articles/PMC1856434.
6. Wu, S., Yi, J., Zhang, Y. G., Zhou, J., Sun, J. "Leaky intestine and impaired microbiome in an amyotrophic lateral sclerosis mouse model." *Physiol Rep*. 2015, Apr 3; (4).
7. Bekkering, P., Jafri, I., van Overveld, F. J., Rijkers, G. T. "The intricate association between gut microbiota and development of type 1, type 2 and type 3 diabetes." *Expert Rev Clin Immunol*. 2013, Nov 9; (11):1031–41.

8. Kelly, J. R., et al. "Breaking down the barriers: the gut microbiome, intestinal permeability and stress-related psychiatric disorders." *Front Cell Neurosci.* 2015, Oct 14; 9:392.

9. Vojdani, A., Vojdani, C. "Immune reactivity to food coloring." *Altern Ther Health Med.* 2015; 21 Suppl 1:52–62.

10. Julio-Pieper, M., Bravo, J. A., Aliaga, E., Gotteland, M. "Review article: intestinal barrier dysfunction and central nervous system disorders—a controversial association." *Aliment Pharmacol Ther.* 2014, Nov; 40(10):1187–201.

11. Mosci, P., et al. "Involvement of IL-17A in preventing the development of deep-seated candidiasis from oropharyngeal infection." *Microbes Infect.* 2014, Aug 16; (8):678–89.

12. Camilleri, M., et al. "Intestinal barrier function in health and gastrointestinal disease." *Neurogastroenterol Motil.* 2012, Jun 24; (6):503–12.

13. Maes, M., Mihaylova, I., Leunis, J. C. "Increased serum IgA and IgM against LPS of enterobacteria in chronic fatigue syndrome (CFS): indication for the involvement of gram-negative enterobacteria in the etiology of CFS and for the presence of an increased gut-intestinal permeability." *J Affect Disord.* 2007, Apr; 99(1–3):237–40. Epub. 2006, Sep 27.

14. Merga, Y., Campbell, B. J., Rhodes, J. M. "Mucosal barrier, bacteria and inflammatory bowel disease: possibilities for therapy." *Dig Dis.* 2014; 32(4):475–83.

15. Goebel, A., et al. "Altered intestinal permeability in patients with primary fibromyalgia and in patients with complex regional pain syndrome." *Rheumatology* (Oxford). 2008, Aug; 47(8):1223–27.

16. Lacy, B. E., Chey, W. D., Lembo, A. J. "New and Emerging Treatment Options for Irritable Bowel Syndrome." *Gastroenterol Hepatol* (NY). 2015, Apr 11; (4 Suppl 2):1–19.

17. Bardella, M. T., et al. "Autoimmune disorders in patients affected by celiac sprue and inflammatory bowel disease." *Ann Med.* 2009; 41(2):139–43.

18. Camilleri, M., et al. "Intestinal barrier function in health and gastrointestinal disease." *Neurogastroenterol Motil.* 2012, Jun 24; (6):503–12.

19. Fresko, I., et al. "Intestinal permeability in Behçet's syndrome." *Ann Rheum Dis.* 2001, Jan; 60(1):65–66.

20. Gérard, P. "Gut microbiota and obesity." *Cell Mol Life Sci.* 2015, Oct 12.

21. De Roos, N. M., et al. "The effects of the multispecies probiotic mixture Ecologic Barrier on migraine: results of an open-label pilot study." *Benef Microbes.* 2015, Oct 15; 6(5):641–6.

22. Nouri, M., et al. "Intestinal barrier dysfunction develops at the onset of experimental autoimmune encephalomyelitis, and can be induced by adoptive transfer of auto-reactive T cells." *PLoS One.* 2014, Sep 3; 9(9):e106335.

23. Brenner, D. A., Paik, Y. H., Schnabl, B. "Role of Gut Microbiota in Liver Disease." *J Clin Gastroenterol.* 2015, Nov–Dec; 49 Suppl 1:S25–27.

24. Forsyth, C. B., et al. "Increased intestinal permeability correlates with sigmoid mucosa alpha-synuclein staining and endotoxin exposure markers in early Parkinson's disease." *PLoS One.* Dec 2011; 6(12):e28032.

25. Zhang, D., et al. "Serum zonulin is elevated in women with polycystic ovary syndrome and correlates with insulin resistance and severity of anovulation." *Eur J Endocrinol.* 2015, Jan; 172(1):29–36.

26. Galland, L. "The gut microbiome and the brain." *J Med Food.* 2014, Dec 17; (12):1261–72. doi: 10.1089/jmf.2014.7000. Review. PubMed PMID: 25402818; PubMed Central PMCID: PMC4259177.

27. Lerner, A., Matthias, T. "Rheumatoid arthritis-celiac disease relationship: Joints get that gut feeling." *Autoimmun Rev.* 2015, Nov 14; (11):1038–47.

28. Pike, M. G., et al. "Increased intestinal permeability in atopic eczema." *J Invest Dermatol.* 1986, Feb; 86(2):101–4. PubMed PMID: 3745938; Humbert, P., Bidet, A., Treffel, P., Drobacheff, C., Agache, P. "Intestinal permeability in patients with psoriasis." *J Dermatol Sci.* 1991, Jul 2; (4):324–6. PubMed PMID: 1911568.

29. Li, X., Atkinson, M. A. "The role for gut permeability in the pathogenesis of type 1 diabetes—a solid or leaky concept?" *Pediatr Diabetes.* 2015, Nov 16; (7):485–92.

30. Vaarala, O., Atkinson, M. A., Neu, J. "The 'Perfect Storm' for Type 1 Diabetes: The Complex Interplay Between Intestinal Microbiota, Gut Permeability, and Mucosal Immunity." *Diabetes.* 2008; 57(10):2555–62. doi: 10.2337/db08-0331.

31. Gomes, J. M., Costa, J. A., Alfenas, R. C. "Could the beneficial effects of dietary calcium on obesity and diabetes control be mediated by changes in intestinal microbiota and integrity?" *Br J Nutr.* 2015, Dec; 114(11):1756–65.

32. Prager, M., Buettner, J., Buening, C. "Genes involved in regulation of intestinal permeability and their role in ulcerative colitis." *J Dig Dis.* 2015 Oct 29.

33. Bouchaud, G., et al. "Consecutive Food and Respiratory Allergies Amplify Systemic and Gut but Not Lung Outcomes in Mice." *J Agric Food Chem.* 2015, Jul 22; 63(28):6475–83.

34. Fasano, A. "Zonulin and its regulation of intestinal barrier function: the biological door to inflammation, autoimmunity, and cancer." *Physiol Rev.* 2011, Jan; 91(1):151–75.

35. www.mountsinai.org/patient-care/service-areas/children/areas-of-care/childrens-environmental-health-center/childrens-disease-and-the-environment/children-and-toxic-chemicals.

36. www.cdc.gov/drugresistance/threat-report-2013.

37. Dethlefsen, L., Relman, D. A. "Incomplete recovery and individualized responses of the human distal gut microbiota to repeated antibiotic perturbation." *Proc Natl Acad Sci USA.* 2011, Mar 15; 108 Suppl 1:4554–61. doi: 10.1073/pnas.1000087107. *Epub.* 2010, Sep 16.

CHAPTER 2

1. Mind-altering microbes: How the microbiome affects brain and behavior: Elaine Hsiao at TEDxCaltech. www.youtube.com/watch?v=FWT _BLVOASI.
2. Aagaard, K., Ma, J., Antony, K. M., Ganu, R., Petrosino, J., Versalovic, J. "The placenta harbors a unique microbiome." *Sci Transl Med.* 2014, May 21; 6(237):237ra65.
3. http://learn.genetics.utah.edu/content/microbiome/changing/.
4. Centers for Disease Control and Prevention. Threat Report 2013. Antibiotic/Antimicrogial Resistance. www.cdc.gov/drugresistance/threat-report -2013.
5. Schnirring, L. "CDC: Antibiotic-resistant bugs sicken 2 million a year." *CIDRAP News.* 2013, Sept 16. www.cidrap.umn.edu/news-perspective /2013/09/cdc-antibiotic-resistant-bugs-sicken-2-million-year.
6. www.cdc.gov/HAI/organisms/cdiff/Cdiff_infect.html.
7. www.iihs.org/iihs/topics/t/general-statistics/fatalityfacts/overview-of-fatality -facts.
8. www.cdc.gov/nchs/fastats/injury.htm.
9. Le Chatelier, E., et al. "Richness of human gut microbiome correlates with metabolic markers." *Nature.* 2013, Aug 29; 500(7464):541–6.
10. Sheridan, K. "Remote Amazonian Tribe Resistant to Modern Antibiotics." *Sydney Morning Herald.* 2015, April 21. www.smh.com.au/world/remote -amazonian-tribe-resistant-to-modern-antibiotics-20150420-1mpeo2.htm=z.
11. Doucleff, M. "How Modern Life Depletes Our Gut Microbes." www.npr.org /blogs/goatsandsoda/2015/04/21/400393756/how-modern-life-depletes-our -gut-microbes.
12. Gibbons, A. "Resistance to Antibiotics Found in Isolated Amazonian Tribe." *Science.* 2015, April 17.
13. Hehemann, J. H., Correc, G., Barbeyron, T., Helbert, W., Czjzek, M., Michel, G. "Transfer of carbohydrate-active enzymes from marine bacteria to Japanese gut microbiota." *Nature.* 2010, Apr 8; 464(7290):908–12.
14. www.niddk.nih.gov/health-information/health-topics/Anatomy/your-diges tive-system/Pages/anatomy.aspx.
15. Wang, W. L., Lu, R. L., DiPierro, M., Fasano, A. "Zonula occludin toxin, a microtubule binding protein." *World J Gastroenterol.* 2000, Jun; 6(3):330–34.
16. Fasano, A. "Zonulin and its regulation of intestinal barrier function: The

biological door to inflammation, autoimmunity, and cancer." *Physiol Rev.* 2011, Jan; 91(1):151–75.

17. Fasano, A. "Intestinal permeability and its regulation by zonulin: diagnostic and therapeutic implications." *Clin Gastroenterol Hepatol.* 2012, Oct 10 (10):1096–100.

CHAPTER 3

1. Van Cleave, J., Gortmaker, S. L., Perrin, J. M. "Dynamics of obesity and chronic health conditions among children and youth." *JAMA.* 2010, Feb 17; 303(7):623–30.

2. O'Brien, K. "Should we all go gluten free?" *New York Times.* 2011, Nov 25. www.nytimes.com/2011/11/27/magazine/Should-We-All-Go-Gluten-Free .html.

3. Tuomilehto, J. "The emerging global epidemic of type 1 diabetes." *Curr Diab Rep.* 2013, Dec 13; (6):795–804.

4. http://www.foodallergy.org/document.doc?id=194.

5. Jackson, K., et al. "Trends in Allergic Conditions among Children: United States, 1997–2011." *National Center for Health Statistics Data Brief.* 2013. Retrieved from www.cdc.gov/nchs/data/databriefs/db10.htm.

6. Ackerman, J. "The ultimate social network." *Scientific American.* 2012; 306,36–43. Published online: 2012, May 15 doi:10.1038/scientificamerican 0612-36

7. Visser, J., et al. "Tight Junctions, Intestinal Permeability, and Autoimmunity Celiac Disease and Type 1 Diabetes Paradigms." *Annals of the New York Academy of Sciences.* 2009; 1165:195–205. doi:10.1111/j.1749-6632.2009.04037.x.

8. Cox, L. M., et al. "Altering the intestinal microbiota during a critical developmental window has lasting metabolic consequences." *Cell.* 2014, Aug 14; 158(4):705–21.

9. Radano, M. C., et al. "Cesarean section and antibiotic use found to be associated with eosinophilic esophagitis." *J Allergy Clin Immunol Pract.* 2014, Jul–Aug; 2(4):475–477.e1.

10. www.mayoclinic.org/diseases-conditions/eosinophilic-esophagitis/basics /definition/con-20035681.

11. Fasano, A. "Intestinal permeability and its regulation by zonulin: diagnostic and therapeutic implications." *Clin Gastroenterol Hepatol.* 2012, Oct 10; (10):1096–100.

12. Barbaro, M. R., et al. "The role of zonulin in non-celiac gluten sensitivity and irritable bowel syndrome." *Abstract presented at the 23rd United European Gastroenterology Week (UEG Week 2015),* 2015, Oct 24–27, Barcelona, Spain; Fasano, A. Ann. *NY Acad Sci.* 2012; 1258:25–33.

13. Vaarala, O., Atkinson, M. A., Neu, J. "The 'Perfect Storm' for Type 1 Diabe-

tes: The Complex Interplay Between Intestinal Microbiota, Gut Permeability, and Mucosal Immunity." *Diabetes.* 2008; 57(10):2555–62. doi: 10.2337 /db08-0331.

14. Fasano, A. "Intestinal permeability and its regulation by zonulin: diagnostic and therapeutic implications." *Clin Gastroenterol Hepatol.* 2012, Oct 10; (10):1096–100.

15. Fasano, A. "Leaky gut and autoimmune diseases." *Clin Rev Allergy Immunol.* 2012, Feb; 42(1):71–78.

16. http://www.arthritis.org/about-arthritis/types/rheumatoid-arthritis/causes .php.

17. Scher, J. U., Abramson, S. B. "The microbiome and rheumatoid arthritis." *Nat Rev Rheumatol.* 2011, Aug 23; 7(10):569–78.

18. Toivanen, P. "Normal intestinal microbiota in the aetiopathogenesis of rheumatoid arthritis." *Ann Rheum Dis.* 2003, Sep; 62(9):807–11. Review.

19. Ebringer, A., Rashid, T., Wilson, C. "Rheumatoid arthritis, Proteus, anti-CCP antibodies and Karl Popper." *Autoimmun Rev.* 2010 Feb; 9(4):216–23.

20. Laws, P., Barton, A., Warren, R. B. "Psoriatic arthritis—what the dermatologist needs to know." *J. Eur. Acad. Dermatol. Venereol.* 2010; 24(11),1270–77.

21. Wu, J. J., Nguyen, T. U., Poon, K. Y., Herrinton, L. J. "The association of psoriasis with autoimmune diseases." *J Am Acad Dermatol.* 2012, Nov; 67(5):924–30.

22. Menter, A., Gottlieb, A., Feldman, S. R., Van Voorhees, A. S., Leonardi, C. L., Gordon, K. B., Lebwohl, M., Koo, J. Y., Elmets, C. A., Korman, N. J., Beutner, K. R., Bhushan, R. "Guidelines of care for the management of psoriasis and psoriatic arthritis: Section 1. Overview of psoriasis and guidelines of care for the treatment of psoriasis with biologics." *J Am Acad Dermatol.* 2008, May; 58(5):826–50.

23. Hébert, H. L., Ali, F. R., Bowes, J., Griffiths, C. E., Barton, A., Warren, R. B. "Genetic susceptibility to psoriasis and psoriatic arthritis: implications for therapy." *Br. J. Dermatol.* 2012; 166(3),474–82.

24. Tsoi, L. C., Spain, S. L., Knight, J., et al. "Identification of 15 new psoriasis susceptibility loci highlights the role of innate immunity." *Nat. Genet.* 2012; 44(12),1341–48.

25. Capone, K. A., Dowd, S. E., Stamatas, G. N., Nikolovski, J. "Diversity of the human skin microbiome early in life." *J Invest Dermatol.* 2011, Oct; 131(10):2026–32. doi: 10.1038/jid.2011.168. Epub. 2011, Jun 23.

26. Marzano, A. V., et al. "Association of pyoderma gangrenosum, acne, and suppurative hidradenitis (PASH) shares genetic and cytokine profiles with other autoinflammatory diseases." *Medicine* (Baltimore). 2014, Dec; 93(27):e187.

27. Gao, Z., Tseng, C. H., Strober, B. E., Pei, Z., Blaser, M. J. "Substantial altera-

tions of the cutaneous bacterial biota in psoriatic lesions." *PLoS One*. 2008, Jul 23; 3(7):e2719.

28. Capone, K. A., Dowd, S. E., Stamatas, G. N., Nikolovski, J. "Diversity of the human skin microbiome early in life." *J Invest Dermatol*. 2011, Oct; 131(10):2026–32. doi: 10.1038/jid.2011.168. Epub. 2011, Jun 23.

29. Fasano, A. "Leaky gut and autoimmune diseases." *Clin Rev Allergy Immunol*. 2012, Feb; 42 (1):71–78.

30. Fasano, A. "Intestinal permeability and its regulation by zonulin: diagnostic and therapeutic implications." *Clin Gastroenterol Hepatol*. 2012, Oct 10; (10):1096–100.

31. Aguilar, M., Bhuket, T., Torres, S., Liu, B., Wong, R. J. "Prevalence of the Metabolic Syndrome in the United States, 2003–2012." *JAMA*, 2015; 313(19):1973.

32. Fasano, A. "Leaky gut and autoimmune diseases." *Clin Rev Allergy Immunol*. 2012, Feb; 42(1):71–78.

33. De Magistris, L., et al. "Alterations of the intestinal barrier in patients with autism spectrum disorders and in their first-degree relatives." *J Pediatr Gastroenterol Nutr*. 2010, Oct; 51(4):418–24.

34. Fasano, A. "Zonulin and its regulation of intestinal barrier function: the biological door to inflammation, autoimmunity, and cancer." *Physiol Rev*. 2011, Jan; 91(1):151–75.

CHAPTER 4

1. Afshinnekoo, E., et al. "Geospatial Resolution of Human and Bacterial Diversity with City-Scale Metagenomics." *Cell Systems*. 2015, July 29; 1(1): 72–87

2. Brodwin, E. "A Geneticist Says Any New Parent Should 'Roll Their Child on the Floor of the New York Subway'—Here's Why." *Business Insider*. 2015, August 15. www.businessinsider.com/what-is-the-hygiene-hypothesis -2015-8.

3. Ackerman, J. "The ultimate social network." *Scientific American*. 2012; 306,36–43. Published online: 2012, May 15. doi:10.1038/scientificamerican 0612-36.

4. Callahan, G. N. "Eating Dirt." *Emerging Infectious Diseases*. Centers for Disease Control and Prevention;" 9:8; 2003, Aug. wwwnc.cdc.gov/eid/article /9/8/03-0033.

5. Nielsen, F. H. "Ultratrace Minerals." (Williams & Wilkins, 1999). Permanent URL: http://naldc.nal.usda.gov/catalog/46493.

6. Amaranthus, M. and Allyn, B. "Healthy Soil Microbes Healthy People." *The Atlantic*. 2013, Jun 11. www.theatlantic.com/health/archive/2013/06 /healthy-soil-microbes-healthy-people/276710/?single_page=true.

7. Hesselmar, B., Hicke-Roberts, A., Wennergren, G. "Allergy in children in hand versus machine dishwashing." *Pediatrics*. 2015 Mar; 135(3):e590–7.
8. Callahan, G. N. "Eating Dirt." *Emerging Infectious Diseases*. Centers for Disease Control and Prevention. 2003; 9(8). Aug wwwnc.cdc.gov/eid /article/9/8/03-0033.
9. Wexler, H. M. "Bacteroides: the Good, the Bad, and the Nitty-Gritty." *Clinical Microbiology Reviews*. 2007; 20(4):593–621. doi:10.1128/CMR.00008-07.
10. Hertzler, S. R., Clancy, S. M. "Kefir improves lactose digestion and tolerance in adults with lactose maldigestion." *J Am Diet Assoc*. 2003 May; 103(5):582–7.
11. Küpeli, A. E., Orhan, D. D., Gürbüz, I., Yesilada, E. "In vivo activity assessment of a 'honey-bee pollen mix' formulation." *Pharm Biol*. 2010 Mar; 48(3):253–9.
12. Wegienka, G., et al. "Lifetime dog and cat exposure and dog- and cat-specific sensitization at age 18 years." *Clin Exp Allergy*. 2011, Jul; 41(7):979–86.
13. Katz, U., Shoenfeld, Y., Zakin, V., Sherer, Y., Sukenik, S. "Scientific evidence of the therapeutic effects of dead sea treatments: a systematic review." *Semin Arthritis Rheum*. 2012, Oct; 42(2):186–200. doi: 10.1016/j.semarthrit .2012.02.006.

CHAPTER 5

1. Winzell, M. S., Ahrén, B. "The high-fat diet-fed mouse: a model for studying mechanisms and treatment of impaired glucose tolerance and type 2 diabetes." *Diabetes*. 2004, Dec; 53 Suppl 3:S215-9.
2. O'Keefe, S. J., et al. "Fat, fibre and cancer risk in African Americans and rural Africans." *Nat Commun*. 2015, Apr 28; 6:6342.
3. Spector, T. "Your Gut Bacteria Don't Like Junk Food—Even If You Do." *The Conversation*, 2015, May 10. https://theconversation.com/your-gut-bacteria -dont-like-junk-food-even-if-you-do-41564.
4. Lerner, A., Matthias, T. "Changes in intestinal tight junction permeability associated with industrial food additives explain the rising incidence of autoimmune disease." *Autoimmun Rev*. 2015, Jun 14; (6):479–89.
5. Esmaillzadeh, A., Azadbakht, L. "Home use of vegetable oils, markers of systemic inflammation, and endothelial dysfunction among women." *Am J Clin Nutr*. 2008, Oct; 88(4):913–21.
6. Santarelli, R. L., Pierre, F., Corpet, D. E. "Processed meat and colorectal cancer: a review of epidemiologic and experimental evidence." *Nutr Cancer*. 2008; 60(2):131–44.
7. Esmaillzadeh, A., Azadbakht, L. "Home use of vegetable oils, markers of systemic inflammation, and endothelial dysfunction among women." *Am J Clin Nutr*. 2008, Oct; 88(4):913–21.

8. Azzouz, A., Jurado-Sánchez, B., Souhail, B., Ballesteros, E. "Simultaneous determination of 20 pharmacologically active substances in cow's milk, goat's milk, and human breast milk by gas chromatography–mass spectrometry." *J Agric Food Chem.* 2011, May 11; 59(9):5125–32. doi: 10.1021/jf200364w. Epub 2011 Apr 15.

9. Harkinson, J. "You're drinking the wrong kind of milk." *Mother Jones.* 2014, Mar 12. www.motherjones.com/environment/2014/03/a1-milk-a2-milk-america.

10. van der Hulst, R. R., van Kreel, B. K., von Meyenfeldt, M. F., Brummer, R. J., Arends, J. W., Deutz, N. E., Soeters, P. B. "Glutamine and the preservation of gut integrity." *Lancet.* 1993, May 29; 341(8857):1363–5.

11. Punzi, J. S., Lamont, M., Haynes, D., Epstein, R. L., "USDA Pesticide Data Program: Pesticide Residues on Fresh and Processed Fruit and Vegetables, Grains, Meats, Milk, and Drinking Water." *Outlooks on Pesticide Management.* 2005, June.

12. Behall, K. M., Scholfield, D. J., Yuhaniak, I., Canary, J. "Diets containing high amylose vs amylopectin starch: effects on metabolic variables in human subjects." *Am J Clin Nutr.* 1989, Feb; 49(2):337–44.

13. Ciacci, C., et al. "Effect of beta-glucan, inositol and digestive enzymes in GI symptoms of patients with IBS." *Eur Rev Med Pharmacol Sci.* 2011, Jun; 15(6):637–43.

14. Korponay-Szabo, I. R., et al. "Food-grade gluten degrading enzymes to treat dietary transgressions in coeliac adolescents." *Journal of Pediatric Gastroenterology and Nutrition;* 43rd Annual Meeting of ESPGHAN; Istanbul. 2010. p. E68. 2010.

15. Trinidad. T. P., Loyola, A. S., Mallillin, A. C., Valdez, D. H., Askali, F. C., Castillo, J. C., Resaba, R. L., Masa, D. B. "The cholesterol-lowering effect of coconut flakes in humans with moderately raised serum cholesterol." *J Med Food.* 2004, Summer; 7(2):136–40.

16. Sategna-Guidetti, C., Bruno, M., Mazza, E., Carlino, A., Predebon, S., Tagliabue, M., Brossa, C. "Autoimmune thyroid diseases and coeliac disease." *Eur J Gastroenterol Hepatol.* 1998, Nov 10; (11):927–31.

17. Dontas, A. S., Zerefos, N. S., Panagiotakos, D. B., Vlachou, C., Valis, D. A. "Mediterranean diet and prevention of coronary heart disease in the elderly." *Clin Interv Aging.* 2007; 2(1):109–15. Review. Erratum in: *Clin Interv Aging.* 2008; 3(2):397.

18. http://umm.edu/health/medical/altmed/supplement/flaxseed-oil.

19. de Kort, S., Keszthelyi, D., Masclee, A. A. "Leaky gut and diabetes mellitus: What is the link?" *Obes Rev.* 2011, Jun; 12(6):449–58.

20. Yang, Q., et al. "Added sugar intake and cardiovascular diseases mortality

among US adults." *JAMA Intern Med.* 2014 Apr; 174(4):516–24. doi: 10.1001 /jamainternmed.2013.13563.

21. United States Department of Agriculture, Economic Research Service. (2012). USDA Sugar Supply: Tables 51–53: US Consumption of Caloric Sweeteners. Retrieved from http://www.ers.usda.gov/data-products/sugar -and-sweeteners-yearbook-tables.aspx.

22. http://www.agmrc.org/commodities__products/livestock/bees-profile/.

23. Schneider, A. "Tests Show More Store Honey Isn't Honey." *Food Safety News.* 2011, Nov 7. http://www.foodsafetynews.com/2011/11/tests-show -most-store-honey-isnt-honey/.

24. Allen, K. L., Molan, P. C., Reid, G. M. "A survey of the antibacterial activity of some New Zealand honeys." *J Pharm Pharmacol.* 1991, Dec; 43(12): 817–22.

25. Ferdman, R. "Where people around the world eat the most sugar and fat." *Washington Post.* 2015, Feb 5. https://www.washingtonpost.com/news /wonk/wp/2015/02/05/where-people-around-the-world-eat-the-most-sugar -and-fat/.

26. Proverbs 25:6 NIV.

27. Swithers, S. E. "Artificial sweeteners produce the counterintuitive effect of inducing metabolic derangements." *Trends Endocrinol Metab.* 2013 Sep; 24(9):431–41.

28. Schiffman, S. S., Rother, K. I. "Sucralose, a synthetic organochlorine sweetener: overview of biological issues." *J Toxicol Environ Health B Crit Rev.* 2013; 16(7):399–451.

29. Abou-Donia, M. B., El-Masry, E. M., Abdel-Rahman, A. A., McLendon, R. E., Schiffman, S. S. "Splenda alters gut microflora and increases intestinal p-glycoprotein and cytochrome p-450 in male rats." *J Toxicol Environ Health A.* 2008; 71(21):1415–29.

30. Nettleton, J. A., et al. "Diet soda intake and risk of incident metabolic syndrome and type 2 diabetes in the Multi-Ethnic Study of Atherosclerosis (MESA)." *Diabetes Care.* 2009, Apr; 32(4):688–94.

CHAPTER 6

1. Olszak, T., An, D., Zeissig, S., Vera, M. P., Richter, J., Franke, A., Glickman, J. N., Siebert, R., Baron, R. M., Kasper, D. L., Blumberg, R. S. "Microbial exposure during early life has persistent effects on natural killer T cell function." *Science.* 2012, Apr 27; 336(6080):489–93.

2. Khazan, O. "How Often People in Various Countries Shower." *Atlantic Monthly.* 2015, Feb 17. www.theatlantic.com/health/archive/2015/02/how -often-people-in-various-countries-shower/385470.

3. Scott, J. "My No-Soap, No-Shampoo, Bacteria-Rich Hygiene Experiment."

New York Times. 2014, May 22. http://www.nytimes.com/2014/05/25 /magazine/my-no-soap-no-shampoo-bacteria-rich-hygiene-experiment.html.

4. Spak, C. J., et al. "Tissue response of gastric mucosa after ingestion of fluoride." *BMJ: British Medical Journal.* 1989; 298(6689):1686–87.

5. Mandel, D. R., Eichas, K., Holmes, J. "Bacillus coagulans: a viable adjunct therapy for relieving symptoms of rheumatoid arthritis according to a randomized, controlled trial." *BMC Complement Altern Med.* 2010, Jan 12; 10:1.

6. Kumar, R., et al. "Cordyceps sinensis promotes exercise endurance capacity of rats by activating skeletal muscle metabolic regulators." *J Ethnopharmacol.* 2011, Jun 14; 136(1):260–6.

7. Suarez-Arroyo, I. J., et al. "Anti-tumor effects of Ganoderma lucidum (reishi) in inflammatory breast cancer in in vivo and in vitro models." *PLoS One.* 2013; 8(2):e57431.

8. Liao, S. F., et al. "Immunization of fucose-containing polysaccharides from Reishi mushroom induces antibodies to tumor-associated Globo H-series epitopes." *Proc Natl Acad Sci USA.* 2013, Aug 20; 110(34):13809–14.

9. Patel, S., Goyal, A. "Recent developments in mushrooms as anti-cancer therapeutics: a review." *3 Biotech.* 2012, Mar; 2(1):1–15.

10. Wong, J. Y., et al. "Gastroprotective Effects of Lion's Mane Mushroom Hericium erinaceus (Bull.:Fr.) Pers. (Aphyllophoromycetideae) Extract against Ethanol-Induced Ulcer in Rats." *Evid Based Complement Alternat Med.* 2013; 2013:492976.

11. Torkelson, C. J., Sweet, E., Martzen, M. R., Sasagawa, M., Wenner, C. A., Gay, J., Putiri, A., Standish, L. J. "Phase 1 Clinical Trial of Trametes versicolor in Women with Breast Cancer." *ISRN Oncol.* 2012; 2012:251632.

12. Lindequist, U., Niedermeyer, T. H., Jülich, W. D. "The pharmacological potential of mushrooms." *Evid Based Complement Alternat Med.* 2005, Sep; 2(3):285–99.

13. http://umm.edu/health/medical/altmed/supplement/spirulina.

14. https://www.mskcc.org/cancer-care/integrative-medicine/herbs/blue -green-algae.

15. Morita, K., Ogata, M., Hasegawa, T. "Chlorophyll derived from Chlorella inhibits dioxin absorption from the gastrointestinal tract and accelerates dioxin excretion in rats." *Environ Health Perspect.* 2001, Mar 10; 9(3):289–94.

16. Pfaller, M. A., Diekema, D. J. "Epidemiology of invasive candidiasis: a persistent public health problem." *Clin Microbiol Rev.* 2007, Jan; 20(1):133–63. Review.

17. Soltani, M., Khosravi, A. R., Asadi, F., Shokri, H. "Evaluation of protective efficacy of Spirulina platensis in Balb/C mice with candidiasis." *J Mycol Med.* 2012, Dec; 22(4):329–34.

18. Reardon. "Phage Therapy Gets Revitalized." *Nature*. 2014, June 3. http://www.nature.com/news/phage-therapy-gets-revitalized-1.15348.

19. Abedon, S. T., Kuhl, S. J., Blasdel, B. G., Kutter, E. M. "Phage treatment of human infections." *Bacteriophage*. 2011 Mar; 1(2):66–85.

20. Guslandi, M., Giollo, P., Testoni, P. A. "A pilot trial of Saccharomyces boulardii in ulcerative colitis." *Eur J Gastroenterol Hepatol*. 2003, Jun; 15(6):697–8.

21. Castagliuolo, I., Riegler, M. F., Valenick, L., LaMont, J. T., Pothoulakis, C. "Saccharomyces boulardii protease inhibits the effects of Clostridium difficile toxins A and B in human colonic mucosa." *Infect Immun*. 1999, Jan; 67(1):302–7.

22. Buts, J. P., De Keyser, N., De Raedemaeker, L. "Saccharomyces boulardii enhances rat intestinal enzyme expression by endoluminal release of polyamines." *Pediatr Res*. 1994, Oct; 36(4):522–27.

23. Weber, G., Adamczyk, A., Freytag, S. "Treatment of acne with a yeast preparation." *Fortschr Med*. 1989, Sep 10; 107(26):563–6.

24. Visser, S. A. "Effect of humic substances on mitochondrial respiration and oxidative phosphorylation." *Sci Total Environ*. 1987, Apr; 62:347–54.

25. Prudden, J. F. "The biological activity of bovine cartilage preparations." *Seminars in Arthritis and Rheumatology*. Summer 1974, 3(4):287–321.

26. Samonina, G., et al. "Protection of gastric mucosal integrity by gelatin and simple proline-containing peptides." *Pathophysiology*. 2000, Apr; 7(1):69–73.

27. Daniel, K. T. "Why Broth is Beautiful: Essential Roles for Proline, Glycine and Gelatin." Weston A. Price Foundation. http://www.westonaprice.org/food-features/why-broth-is-beautiful (accessed 2013, June 18).

28. Rennard, B. O., et al. "Chicken soup inhibits neutrophil chemotaxis in vitro." *Chest*. 2000, Oct; 118(4):1150–7.

CHAPTER 7

1. Scheer, R. and Moss, D. "Dirt Poor: Have Fruits and Vegetables Become Less Nutritious?" *Scientific American*. 2011, April 27. www.scientificamerican.com/article/soil-depletion-and-nutrition-loss.

2. Jack, A. "Nutrition Under Siege." *One Peaceful World* (Kushi Institute newsletter), Becket, MA, Spring 1998; 1,7–8.

3. Scheer, R. and Moss, D. "Dirt Poor: Have Fruits and Vegetables Become Less Nutritious?" *Scientific American*. 2011, April 27. www.scientificamerican.com/article/soil-depletion-and-nutrition-loss.

4. Marler, J. B., Wallin, J. R. "Human Health, the Nutritional Quality of Harvested Food and Sustainable Farming Systems." *Nutrition Security Institute*. www.nutritionsecurity.org.

5. Scheer, R. and Moss, D. "Dirt Poor: Have Fruits and Vegetables Become Less Nutritious?" *Scientific American*. 2011, April 27. www.scientificamerican.com/article/soil-depletion-and-nutrition-loss.

6. Kötke, W. H. *The Final Empire: The Collapse of Civilization and the Seed of the Future*. (Bloomington, IN: AuthorHouse, 2007).

7. Powell, A. L., Giovannoni, J. "Uniform Ripening Encodes a Golden 2-like Transcription Factor Regulating Tomato Fruit Chloroplast Development." *Science*. 2012, June 29. Vol. 336 no. 6089; 1711–1715; www.sciencemag .org/content/336/6089/1711.

8. Joly Condette, C., et al. "Increased Gut Permeability and Bacterial Translocation after Chronic Chlorpyrifos Exposure in Rats." Blachier, F., ed. *PLoS One*. 2014; 9(7):e102217.

9. www2.epa.gov/ingredients-used-pesticide-products/revised-human-health -risk-assessment-chlorpyrifos.

10. Cressey, D. "Widely Used Herbicide Linked to Cancer." *Nature*. 2015, March 24. www.nature.com/news/widely-used-herbicide-linked-to-cancer -1.17181.

11. Samsel, A., Seneff, S. "Glyphosate, pathways to modern diseases II: Celiac sprue and gluten intolerance." *Interdisciplinary Toxicology*. 2013; 6(4):159– 84. doi:10.2478/intox-2013-0026.

12. Smith, B. "Organic Foods vs Supermarket Foods: Element Levels." *Journal of Applied Nutrition*. 1993; 45:35–39. https://www.organicconsumers.org/ old_articles/Organic/organicstudy.php.

13. Hertzler, S. R., Clancy, S. M. "Kefir Improves Lactose Digestion and Tolerance in Adults with Lactose Maldigestion." *Journal of the American Dietetic Association*. 2003, May; 103(5):582–7.

14. Choi, I. H. "Kimchi, a Fermented Vegetable, Improves Serum Lipid Profiles in Healthy Young Adults." *Journal of Medicinal Food*. 2013, Mar; 16(3):223–9.

15. Sun, P., Wang, J. Q., Zhang, H. T. "Effects of Bacillus subtilis natto on performance and immune function of preweaning calves." *J Dairy Sci*. 2010, Dec; 93(12):5851–5.

16. Koehler, P., Hartmann, G., Wieser, H., Rychlik, M. "Changes of folates, dietary fiber, and proteins in wheat as affected by germination." *J Agric Food Chem*. 2007, Jun 13; 55(12):4678–83.

17. www.ewg.org/key-issues/consumer-products/cosmetics.

18. Barry, R. *The Melaleuca Wellness Guide*. Ed. Richard M. Barry. RM Barry Publications. 2011.

19. Braoudaki, M., Hilton, A. C. "Adaptive resistance to biocides in Salmonella enterica and Escherichia coli O157 and cross-resistance to antimicrobial agents." *J Clin Microbiol*. 2004, Jan; 42(1):73–78.

CHAPTER 8

1. Kelly, J. R., Kennedy, P. J., Cryan, J. F., Dinan, T. G., Clarke, G., Hyland, N. P. "Breaking down the barriers: The gut microbiome, intestinal perme-

ability and stress-related psychiatric disorders." *Front Cell Neurosci.* 2015, Oct 14; 9:392.

2. Alcock, J., Maley, C. C., Aktipis, C. A. "Is eating behavior manipulated by the gastrointestinal microbiota? Evolutionary pressures and potential mechanisms." *Bioessays.* 2014, Oct; 36(10):940–99.

3. Vanuystel, T., et al. "Psychological Stress and Corticotropin-Releasing Hormones Increase Intestinal Permeability in Humans by a Mast Cell-Dependent Mechanism." *Gut.* 2014; 63:1293–99. http://gut.bmj.com/content/63/8/1293.short.

4. Vanuytsel, T., van Wanrooy, S., Vanheel, H., Vanormelingen, C., Verschueren, S., Houben, E., Salim Rasoel, S., Tóth, J., Holvoet, L., Farré, R., Van Oudenhove, L., Boeckxstaens, G., Verbeke, K., Tack, J. "Psychological stress and corticotropin-releasing hormone increase intestinal permeability in humans by a mast cell-dependent mechanism." *Gut.* 2014, Aug; 63(8):1293–9.

5. Puri, H. S. *Rasayana: ayurvedic herbs for longevity and rejuvenation— Volume 2 of Traditional herbal medicines for modern times.* s.l.: CRC Press, 2002

6. Bested, A. C., Logan, A. C., Selhub, E. M. "Intestinal microbiota, probiotics and mental health: From Metchnikoff to modern advances: Part II— contemporary contextual research." *Gut Pathog.* 2013, Mar 14; 5(1):3.

7. www.takingcharge.csh.umn.edu/explore-healing-practices/food-medicine / why-being-mindful-matters.

8. Alcock, J., Maley, C. C., Aktipis, C. A. "Is eating behavior manipulated by the gastrointestinal microbiota? Evolutionary pressures and potential mechanisms." *Bioessays.* 2014, Oct; 36(10):940–49.

9. Sanchez, M., et al. "Effect of Lactobacillus rhamnosus CGMCC1.3724 supplementation on weight loss and maintenance in obese men and women." *Br J Nutr.* 2014, Apr 28; 111(8):1507–19.

10. Bercik, P., Park, A. J., Sinclair, D., Khoshdel, A., Lu, J., Huang, X., Deng, Y., Blennerhassett, P. A., Fahnestock, M., Moine, D., Berger, B., Huizinga, J. D., Kunze, W., McLean, P. G., Bergonzelli, G. E., Collins, S. M., Verdu, E. F. "The anxiolytic effect of Bifidobacterium longum NCC3001 involves vagal pathways for gut-brain communication." *Neurogastroenterol Motil.* 2011, Dec; 23(12):1132–39.

11. Bravo, J. A., Forsythe, P., Chew, M. V., Escaravage, E., Savignac, H. M., Dinan, T. G., Bienenstock, J., Cryan, J. F. "Ingestion of Lactobacillus strain regulates emotional behavior and central GABA receptor expression in a mouse via the vagus nerve." *Proc Natl Acad Sci USA.* 2011, Sep 20; 108(38):16050–55.

12. Anabrees J., Indrio F., Paes B., AlFaleh K. "Probiotics for infantile colic: a systematic review." *BMC Pediatr.* 2013 Nov 15; 13: 186.

13. Tillisch, K., et al. "Consumption of Fermented Milk Product With Probiotic Modulates Brain Activity." *Gastroenterology.* Volume 144; Issue 7; 1394–1401.e4.

14. Schmidt, K., Cowen, P. J., Harmer, C. J., Tzortzis, G., Errington, S., Burnet, P. W. "Prebiotic intake reduces the waking cortisol response and alters emotional bias in healthy volunteers." *Psychopharmacology* (Berl). 2015, May; 232(10):1793–801.

15. Koopman, F. A., Stoof, S. P., Straub, R. H., Van Maanen, M. A., Vervoordeldonk, M. J., Tak, P. P. "Restoring the balance of the autonomic nervous system as an innovative approach to the treatment of rheumatoid arthritis." *Mol Med.* 2011, Sep–Oct; 17(9–10):937–48.

16. www.wisebrain.org/ParasympatheticNS.pdf.

CHAPTER 9

1. Herbert, M. K., Weis, R., Holzer, P. "The enantiomers of tramadol and its major metabolite inhibit peristalsis in the guinea pig small intestine via differential mechanisms." *BMC Pharmacol.* 2007, Mar 16; 7:5.

2. Panchal, S. J., Müller-Schwefe, P., Wurzelmann, J. I. "Opioid-induced bowel dysfunction: prevalence, pathophysiology and burden." *Int J Clin Pract.* 2007, Jul; 61(7): 1181–87.

3. www.nytimes.com/2015/11/08/opinion/sunday/how-doctors-helped-drive-the-addiction-crisis.html.

4. Starfield, B. "Is US health really the best in the world?" *JAMA.* 2000, Jul 26; 284(4):483–5.

5. www.cancer.org/acs/groups/cid/documents/webcontent/002385-pdf.pdf.

6. Van Boeckel, T. P., et al. "Global antibiotic consumption 2000 to 2010: an analysis of national pharmaceutical sales data." *Lancet Infectious Diseases.* 14.8(2014):742–50.

7. www.cdc.gov/media/releases/2015/p0225-clostridium-difficile.html.

8. www.mayoclinic.org/diseases-conditions/c-difficile/basics/causes/con-20029664.

9. Shehab, N., Patel, P. R., Srinivasan, A., Budnitz, D. S. "Emergency department visits for antibiotic-associated adverse events." *Clin Infect Dis.* 2008, Sep 15; 47(6):735–43.

10. Karadsheh, Z., Sule, S. "Fecal transplantation for the treatment of recurrent clostridium difficile infection." *N Am J Med Sci.* 2013, Jun; 5(6):339–43.

11. www.cdc.gov/media/dpk/2013/docs/getsmart/dpk-antibiotics-week-lauri-hicks-audio-transcript.pdf.

12. Hempel, S., et al. "Probiotics for the Prevention and Treatment of Antibiotic-Associated Diarrhea." *Journal of American Medical Association,* 2012; 307(18):1959–1669.

13. Floch, M. H. "Recommendations for Probiotic Use in Humans—a 2014 Update." *Pharmaceuticals.* 2014; 7,999–1007.

14. Woodard, G. A., Encarnacion, B., Downey, J. R., Peraza, J., Chong, K., Hernandez-Boussard, T., Morton, J. M. "Probiotics improve outcomes after Roux-en-Y gastric bypass surgery: A prospective randomized trial." *J Gastrointest Surg.* 2009, Jul; 13(7):1198–204.

15. Smith, T. J., Rigassio-Radler, D., Denmark, R., Haley, T., Touger-Decker, R. "Effect of Lactobacillus rhamnosus LGG® and Bifidobacterium animalis ssp. lactis BB-12® on health-related quality of life in college students affected by upper respiratory infections." *Br J Nutr.* 2013, Jun; 109(11):1999–2007.

16. Steenbergen, L., Sellaro, R., van Hemert, S., Bosch, J. A., Colzato, L. S. "A randomized controlled trial to test the effect of multispecies probiotics on cognitive reactivity to sad mood." *Brain Behav Immun.* 2015, Aug; 48:258–64.

17. Oaklander, M. "Can Probiotics Improve Your Mood?" *Time,* 2015, April 10. http://time.com/3817375/probiotics-depression.

18. Sanchez, M., et al. "Effect of Lactobacillus rhamnosus CGMCC1.3724 supplementation on weight loss and maintenance in obese men and women." *Br J Nutr.* 2014, Apr 28; 111(8):1507–19.

19. Tillisch, K., et al. "Consumption of fermented milk product with probiotic modulates brain activity." *Gastroenterology.* 2013, Jun; 144(7):1394–401, 1401.e1–4.

20. Cribby, S., Taylor, M., Reid, G. "Vaginal microbiota and the use of probiotics." *Interdiscip Perspect Infect Dis.* 2008; 2008:256490.

21. Lamprecht, M., et al. "Probiotic supplementation affects markers of intestinal barrier, oxidation, and inflammation in trained men; a randomized, double-blinded, placebo-controlled trial." *J Int Soc Sports Nutr.* 2012, Sep 20; 9(1):45.

22. Roudsari, M. R., et al. "Health effects of probiotics on the skin." *Crit Rev Food Sci Nutr.* 2015; 55(9):1219–40.

23. Chenoll, E., Casinos, B., Bataller, E., Astals, P., Echevarría, J., Iglesias, J. R., Balbarie, P., Ramón, D., Genovés, S. "Novel probiotic Bifidobacterium bifidum CECT 7366 strain active against the pathogenic bacterium Helicobacter pylori." *Appl Environ Microbiol.* 2011, Feb; 77(4):1335–43.

24. Reddy, B. S., Rivenson, A. "Inhibitory effect of Bifidobacterium longum on colon, mammary, and liver carcinogenesis induced by 2-amino-3-methylimidazo[4,5-f]quinoline, a food mutagen." *Cancer Res.* 1993, Sep 1; 53(17):3914–8.

25. Wada M., et al. "Effects of the enteral administration of Bifidobacterium breve on patients undergoing chemotherapy for pediatric malignancies." *Support Care Cancer.* 2010, Jun; 18(6):751–9. doi: 10.1007/s00520-009-0711-6.

26. Whorwell, P. J., et al. "Efficacy of an Encapsulated Probiotic Bifidobacte-

rium Infantis in Women with Irritable Bowel Syndrome." *American Journal of Gastroenterology.* 101(7)1581–90.

27. McFarland, L. V. "Evidence-based review of probiotics for antibiotic-associated diarrhea and Clostridium difficile infections." *Anaerobe.* 2009, Dec; 15(6):274–80.

28. Anderson, J. W., Gilliland, S. E. "Effect of fermented milk (yogurt) containing Lactobacillus acidophilus L1 on serum cholesterol in hypercholesterolemic humans." *J Am Coll Nutr.* 1999, Feb; 18(1):43–50.

29. Raz, R., Stamm, W. E. "A controlled trial of intravaginal estriol in postmenopausal women with recurrent urinary tract infections." *N Engl J Med.* 1993, Sep 9; 329(11):753–6.

30. Bravo, J. A., et al. "Ingestion of Lactobacillus strain regulates emotional behavior and central GABA receptor expression in a mouse via the vagus nerve." *Proc Natl Acad Sci USA.* 2011, Sep 20; 108(38):16050–55.

31. Ciprandi, G., et al. "In vitro effects of Bacillus subtilis on the immune response." *Chemioterapia.* 1986, Dec; 5(6):404–7.

32. Shylakhovenko, V. A. "Anticancer and Immunostimulatory Effects of Nucleoprotein Fraction of Bacillus subtilis." *Experimental Oncology.* 2003, June 25; 119–123.

33. Mandel, D. R., Eichas, K., Holmes, J. "Bacillus coagulans: A viable adjunct therapy for relieving symptoms of rheumatoid arthritis according to a randomized, controlled trial." *BMC Complement Altern Med.* 2010, Jan 12; 10:1.

34. Guslandi, M., Giollo, P., Testoni, P. A. "A pilot trial of Saccharomyces boulardii in ulcerative colitis." *Eur J Gastroenterol Hepatol.* 2003, Jun; 15(6):697–98.

35. Castagliuolo, I., Riegler, M. F., Valenick, L., LaMont, J. T., Pothoulakis, C. "Saccharomyces boulardii protease inhibits the effects of Clostridium difficile toxins A and B in human colonic mucosa." *Infect Immun.* 1999, Jan; 67(1):302–7.

36. Buts, J. P., De Keyser, N., De Raedemaeker, L. "Saccharomyces boulardii enhances rat intestinal enzyme expression by endoluminal release of polyamines." *Pediatr Res.* 1994, Oct; 36(4):522–27.

37. Braden, R., et al. "The Use of the Essential Oil Lavandin to Reduce Preoperative Anxiety in Surgical Patients." *Perianesthesia Nursing.* 24,348–55.

38. Burns, E. E., et al. "An Investigation into the Use of Aromatherapy in Intrapartum Midwifery Practice." *Journal of Alternative and Complementary Medicine.* 2000, April; 6(2):141–47.

CHAPTER 10

1. Bergsson, G., Arnfinnsson, J., Steingrímsson, O., Thormar, H. "In vitro killing of Candida albicans by fatty acids and monoglycerides." *Antimicrob Agents Chemother.* 2001, Nov; 45(11):3209–12.

2. Simopoulos, A. P. "Omega-3 fatty acids in inflammation and autoimmune diseases." *J Am Coll Nutr.* 2002, Dec; 21(6):495–505. Review.

3. Farrukh, A., Mayberry, J. F. "Is there a role for fish oil in inflammatory bowel disease?" *World J Clin Cases.* 2014, Jul 16; 2(7):250–52. doi: 10.12998 /wjcc.v2.i7.250. Review.

4. Vanuytsel, T., et al. "Psychological stress and corticotropin-releasing hormone increase intestinal permeability in humans by a mast cell-dependent mechanism." *Gut.* 2014, Aug; 63(8):1293–99.

5. Field, T. "Massage therapy research review." *Complement Ther Clin Pract.* 2014, Nov; 20(4):224–9. doi: 10.1016/j.ctcp.2014.07.002. Epub. 2014, Aug 1. Review.

6. Karadag, E., et al. "Effects of aromatherapy on sleep quality and anxiety of patients." *Nurs Crit Care.* 2015, Jul 27.

7. Hamilton, J. B., et al. "You need a song to bring you through: the use of religious songs to manage stressful life events." *Gerontologist.* 2013, Feb; 53(1):26–38.

8. Li, Q. "Effect of forest bathing trips on human immune function." *Environ Health Prev Med.* 2010, Jan; 15(1):9–17. doi: 10.1007/s12199-008 -0068-3.

9. Cui, L., et al. "Contribution of a thickened cell wall and its glutamine nonamidated component to the vancomycin resistance expressed by Staphylococcus aureus Mu50." *Antimicrob Agents Chemother.* 2000, Sep; 44(9):2276–85.

10. Catanzaro, D., Rancan, S., Orso, G., Dall'Acqua, S., Brun, P., Giron, M. C., Carrara, M., Castagliuolo, I., Ragazzi, E., Caparrotta, L., Montopoli, M. "Boswellia serrata Preserves Intestinal Epithelial Barrier from Oxidative and Inflammatory Damage." *PLoS One.* 2015. May 8; 10(5):e0125375.

CHAPTER 11

1. Margolin, C. "New Chinese Medicine Tools to Replenish and Repair Our Gut." *Pacific College of Oriental Medicine.* www.pacificcollege.edu/news /blog/2015/05/06/new-chinese-medicine-tools-replenish-and-repair-our -gut.

CHAPTER 12

1. Candida Yeast Infection, Leaky Gut, Irritable Bowel and Food Allergies. Nation Candida Center. www.nationalcandidacenter.com/leaky-gut.

CHAPTER 13

1. Cohen, M. M. "Tulsi (*Ocimum Sanctum*): A Herb for All Reasons." *Journal of Ayurveda and Integrative Medicine.* 2014, Oct–Dec; 5(4):251–259.

CHAPTER 14
1. Candida Yeast Infection, Leaky Gut, Irritable Bowel and Food Allergies. National Candida Center. www.nationalcandidacenter.com/leaky-gut.

CHAPTER 16
1. Everhart, J. E., Khare, M., Hill, M., Maurer, K. R. "Prevalence and ethnic differences in gallbladder disease in the United States." *Gastroenterology.* 1999, Sep; 117(3):632–39.

Index

About the Author

DR. JOSH AXE is a doctor of natural medicine and a clinical nutritionist with a passion to help people get healthy by using food as medicine. He founded one of the largest functional medicine clinics in the United States and runs the popular health website www.draxe.com, where you can find recipes, natural remedies, videos, nutrition advice, and fitness tips. Dr. Axe is a board-certified doctor of natural medicine (DNM), earned his doctorate in chiropractic at Palmer College (DC), and is a certified nutrition specialist (CNS) from the American College of Nutrition. He lives in Nashville, Tennessee, with his wife, Chelsea.